God's Healing Leaves

A User's Guide to Herbology

by Robert McClintock, ND

Printed by:

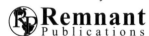

Coldwater, Michigan 49036
www.remnantpublications.com

God's Healing Leaves

This edition published 2013

Copyright © 2013

ISBN 978-1-883012-82-3

TABLE OF CONTENTS

Preface 4

Dedication 6

Kitchen Stuff 7

Combining Herbs 11

Alphabetical listing of Herbs 16

Glossary of terms 84

Useful Abreviations 92

Index 94

The information contained in this book is for educational purposes only. It is not intended to replace sound medical attention or advice. Please do not attempt to use this information to diagnose any diseases. Should you choose to utilize the educational information that is contained herein, you must assume the responsibility of doing so at your own risk.

Why Another Herb Book?

With all of the myriads of books on alternative healing and books on herbology that are on the market today, why would anyone want to write one more? Frankly, I had no intention of ever writing a book. I only compiled the information for my own benefit and my own use. However, when I began teaching classes, and holding seminars about God's gentle medicines around the world, the students would frequently say, "We don't like taking notes! It is a distraction to our learning process, please just let us copy your lecture notes." But my lecture notes were never in such a form that I felt comfortable releasing them to people. As this request was echoed and reechoed with every class, I began to slowly understand that there was a need for yet another book.

What may be unique about this book is corollary to what is unique about the classes and seminars that I have taught throughout the years. The title of the book perhaps reveals the secret, however; let me explain further. As a Christian I believe that God created the universe, our world, and the plants for our use. Yet when I would look in the herbology text books that had been written and compiled thus far, I constantly found that they contained information from spiritualistic or New Age sources. I can only ascribe to Christian theories. I believe that God is our creator and that it is His intention for us to utilize His natural medicines. I do not believe that these plants are here by accident, nor do I believe that they are here due to some mystical positive and negative forces. Throughout the years as I developed this information and compiled it, I filtered out all of this erroneous information. Many of the books lacked specific information about how to use the plants. They would say for a given condition that you had a variety of plants that you could choose from, but rarely did I find specific information about a particular plant with safe doses suggested for that plant. Consequently, I felt motivated to put this information together that I might apply it to my own practice. As I began to use this information and share it in the seminars, I was frequently asked, "Why don't you put this in a book?" I was asked often enough, that in spite of the incredible schedule that I sometimes keep, I have been able to go through and edit the material so that I now feel comfortable in sharing it. I have tried to write the material in such a way that it can be easily understood by the layperson, even those with limited knowledge. I have tried to keep the medical terminology simple and to a minimum.

May the Lord bless you as you explore and put into practice His method of natural healing.

Note:

There are hundreds of medicinal herbs. This book does not cover them all. I have chosen to examine those that are used most frequently or are most easily obtained. You may already enjoy using an herb not covered in this book. Continue to do so if you are comfortable with it.

My Special Thanks!

I want to give a special thanks to my wife Lori, who reluctantly received the job of editing, formating, and doing most of the typing. To all of the people of my class who bought me that wonderful lap top which made this all possible. Also to Marci, who gave me support and made contributions to certain portions of the book. A special thanks to those students and friends for their financial support and for urging me until I finally got off of dead center and got the project done. I would also like to extend an appreciation to my children who see me rather infrequently due to the type of work that I do. Last but not least I would like to give the biggest thanks to the Good Lord for making this information available that I might be able to put it together and attempt to bless and help others.

Robert McClintock

Kitchen Stuff!

The detailed and specific information in this book would be of no practical use if one were not given an introduction to some of the terms with some instruction as how to carry out the specifics in the latter section. Throughout the book you will find many terms that are used over and over. Unless you are familiar with at least a brief overview of how to prepare some of these things, you will find it impossible to actually carry out the instructions that one finds.

I would like to start with some definitions.

Capsules: Many people simply buy pre-encapsulated herbs and pay far more than necessary. Most are unaware that the capsules that they are using are made from animal tissues and generally that of the pig. It is imperative for optimal health especially in these final days of earths history to utilize vegetarian capsules only. These may be obtained from a variety of sources quite freely today. By utilizing a semiautomatic encapsulating device available for approximately $10.00 you may save considerable amounts of money by encapsulating your own herbs.

Decoction: This is herbal tea referred to using the solid parts of plants such as the nuts, roots, rhizomes, barks, seeds and heavy stems. It takes physical action to extract the beneficial properties from these parts of the plant, hence it will take a different action than when making an infusion. To make a decoction we place the plant particles in a pan using 1 teaspoon per cup of water. Bring this to a low simmer for 10-30 minutes. Smaller particles and powders require the least amount of time, larger particles such as shredded barks and roots require the maximum time not to exceed 30 minutes.

Infusion: Infusion is the terminology used to define an herbal tea. But it specifically refers to the parts of the plants that are used and describes a precise method of preparing those parts that will maintain their effectiveness. In making infusions we will be using the aerial or the lighter and upper parts of the plant. These parts contain volatile oils that if not prepared carefully will be damaged or destroyed. These parts may be used in a fresh or dried form. If using a fresh form you will need to use twice as much. Place your herbs, usually 1 teaspoon per cup of water, in a cup, pour boiling water over them, cover the cup and let it steep until cool enough to drink (15-20 minutes). Sometimes we find it necessary to make an infused oil. To make an infused oil place your herbs in a high quality vegetable oil such as olive or corn oil. Place in a glass jar, cover and leave it in the sun for 10-14 days, shaking daily. The sun will cause an extraction process, and will infuse the herb into the oil. At the end of the days you can strain and store the oil preferably in the refrigerator so it does not get rancid. You may accelerate the process by taking your glass jar containing your prospective infused oil, set it in a pan of water with the lid loose on the jar, bring it to a low simmer maintaining this heat for approximately 2 hours. Remove the jar, strain the infusion after it is cool and you will have accelerated greatly the process of making an infused oil.

Infusional-Decoction: Sometimes you will find that it is necessary to combine the effects of the aerial part of one plant with perhaps the bark of another. In doing this you will be making an herbal preparation called an infusional-decoction. You have two choices, you may either make the infusion of the aerial parts of the first plant in one pan and in a separate pan make a decoction of the other. Then mix the two together when they are finished. Occasionally when using this method we find that the volumn of tea is too great to be consumed comfortably, so a second method is prefered.

8

The method that I choose, is to begin with the standard directions for a decoction. Once the decoction has been made and while it is still at the simmering temperature, remove it from the heat, place the aerial parts of the other plant into the already prepared decoction, place a cover over the container and let cool.

Salve: Take your infused oil and melt in some cocoa butter and a small portion of bees wax or paraffin. Allow to cool and the result will be a salve. You will have to experiment with the proportions as they vary with the particular climate that you live in and your own personal preferences. You may extend the life of this product with a natural preservative known as vitamin E oil. Squirt several vitamin E oil capsules into the salve and mix it well, this will help prevent it from becoming racid.

Tinctures: Tinctures are made using vegetable glycerine, alcohol, and sometimes vinegar as extractors and preserving solvents. You will place an herb or blend of herbs into one of these three solutions. Allow it to stand for 10 days, shaking it daily. During that time an extraction has taken place and the beneficial properties of the plant have been leeched into the solution and are suspended. Now strain or purify it and you have a preserved product that may be taken by drops. The reason for using a tincture is to provide an element of ease for traveling. Proper dosages are more readily available and more convenient than when using infusions, decoctions, or capsules. You can just put a few drops into your mouth and the application is finished. They travel well in your pocket, purse or suitcase. You may also evaporate the alcohol off if this has been used, by putting your drops into a cup and pouring boiling water over it and letting it sit for about 10 minutes. The most effective of these solvents is grain alcohol. If you are going to be using it internally make sure that it is not made with rubbing alcohol. It is typically made by home users with Vodka obtained from the liquor store. You may use vegetable glycerine, however; it does not extract as well even though it does store well. The least desirable and effective on the list is vinegar. My preference has been to use grain alcohol for making tinctures. Tinctures may be made in a variety of strengths and manners. I will give you a suggested rule of thumb for making a tincture and you may adapt it to your own liking as you find it necessary. For your first experiment with making a tincture take a one pint jar and put your powdered or cut and sifted plants in it. Pour grain alcohol over the top, stir it until it is thoroughly saturated, making certain that there is excess alcohol covering the herbs so that there is about one inch of clear free alcohol above the plant particles. Place a cover on it and let it stand, shaking it daily for 10 days. You will notice that the plant particles will absorb some of the alcohol and will swell so that your one inch of free space will eventually be diminished by perhaps a half inch. At the end of the 10 days you may strain the entire contents through a muslin cloth. You may find that you may need to wind it tightly and even do some squeezing to extract it all out and not lose any of it. It is recommended that tinctures be stored in amber dropper bottles or jars.

The processes described above are available on an approximately one hour video tape from:

Healing Leaves
P.O. Box 7
Rice, WA. 99167
(509) 738-2177

Combining Herbs

In many books you will find formulas given of herbal combinations that are a little bit confusing. At many health food and supplement stores we find pre-packaged or prepared combinations of herbs that are equally confusing. Frankly, in my years of study of herbology, it has become apparent to me that there are two systems of herbal combining. Number one is called, the "Old wives tale method". Somewhere in the wilds of the frontier, of some unknown there lived the local medicine man or woman. He/she was relied upon by those in his or her community for practical healing. This person either relied upon information that had been handed down to them, or experimented with things on their own for healing. They concocted combinations of plants that were found in their local area through the process of trial, error and experimentation. They were able to discover that beneficial results were obtained in healing by using these combinations. This was an archaic process and many of the herbs contained had nothing to do with the healing. Indeed sometimes the only effect in healing was the placebo effect. Unfortunately, much of what we find in herbal medicine today has been built on the old wives method of herbal formulating.

The second theory of herbal formulation uses a more scientific principle of determining the physical and chemical properties contained in the plant. Then recognizing how they corollate with the physiology of the human body and making a combination of herbs that will produce a desired effect. This latter system is the system that I have come to prefer and use. It is, a much more rational approach to combining herbs. It would take volumes to explain exactly and precisely how this system works, but I can give you a thumbnail sketch that can be the foundation that you may put into practice as you begin to develope your skills along these lines. There are just a couple of basic rules to follow. As you read through the alphabetical listing of herbs contained in this book you will notice that for each herb the physical action is described. Take for instance a refrigerant herb like red raspberry leaf which will help bring about a cooling of a fevered body. It may be combined with perhaps white willow that is an analgesic type herb which should have a similar effect on the body. It would not make sense to combine red raspberry leaf or white willow with the yarrow plant, as the yarrow is a diaphoretic plant which will produce an increase in the body temperature and increase the sweating. These two herbs would have an opposing effect and the net effect would be nothing other than making chaos in the body. This may not lend itself towards good health in the long run. Another rule would be to keep your herbal formulas as simple as possible. Each time you add an herb you add a variety of chemical constituents, and all of these tend to be somewhat confusing to the body if you are blending too many in one combination. It is easier to combine herbs that have been ground into a powder as they lend themselves to being encapsulated much easier. Combining of herbs may be of benefit due to a broadening of the spectrum of effect. Using two or more herbs with similar effects usually produces a stronger effect then one herb on its own. When combining herbs it is sensible to expect to lower the amount of the herbs taken. Example: If you were to take an herb with a dosagel level of 4 caps and another herb with a dosage level of 6 caps you probably not take 10 caps of the combination. You would normally expect to take 4 or 5 caps of the combination.

Harvesting Herbs

Most herbs are at their maximum potency just prior to the plants coming into bloom. It is best to harvest herbs in the morning just after the dew has dried off of the plants, but before the morning sun has gotten hot enough to begin evaporating any of the volitile substances out of the tender parts of the plant.

You may be able to extend your period of time that you can harvest, if the plants that you are harvesting are in the shade.

The plants that you harvest must be prepared properly so that they will keep for long periods of time. It is recommended that you clean all roots, rhizomes, barks, etc. from any soil or animal debrit that may have contaminated them. This may be done with water and a light brissled brush. An old tooth brush works well. It is generally unnecessary to clean the aireal parts of the majority of the plants that we harvest. Once our plants are cleaned it usually works best to chop the heavier parts of the plants apart prior to drying to that they may dry as quickly as possible. This is especially true with heavy roots, nuts, or barks. Areal parts of the plants generally may be dried intact and then chopped or ground into a powder later.

Drying in direct sun light is not recommended. The best method is to dry your plants in an area that is out of the direct sun but has free flowing air and at a higher temperature. Many people dry their plants in the attic of their garage or in a dark room that is warm. Make sure that you lay them out either on a flat tray so that they are not touching one another. Also put them on the tray thin enough so that they have good air flow through them so that they do not mold. The mold or mildew that might accumulate if they are too wet and clumped together will be toxic.

You may also dry in an oven on the lowest setting with the door propped part way open. Some folk find that it works very well to dry in a food drier. All of these methods will work.

Storage

There are many ways to store you herbs but some are better than others. The best way is to store your herbs, once they have been completely dried so that you are certain that they will not mildew or mold, in glass containers that are air tight. Herbs that are stored in dry air tight containers and are stored in a dark cool room will keep will keep for several years. If herbs are not stored in an air tight container and or are stored in direct sunlight will lose their potency after a short period of a few months. It is not necessary to go to the expense of buying dark amber glass. If you have some it will be fine to use it, but it is expensive and you may simply store your herbs in jars such as canning jars or similar type glass jar that you can close tightly. All the amber is for is to keep out the light. You can place your herbs in clear jars and put them in cupboards that have closing doors so that they are stored in the dark. It is essential that they be stored in a room that is fairly cool. It is not recommended to store your herbs in paper or plastic. The paper will allow the volitile substances to evaporate. The plastic, even though it may not allow substances to evaporate from the herbs, there is a potential for the plastic resins to contaminate the herbs that are stored in them. If you have been storing herbs in the proper way and you are afraid that perhaps they may have lost some of their potency, maybe it has been around 3-4 years that you have been storing these things, you have the choice of either throwing them away or determining how much of their potency they may have lost and just taking a larger quantity of the herb to make up for the loss in potency.

A NOTE TO THE READERS:

There are literally hundreds of medicinal plants that you can choose from. The following section contains plants that are predominantly indigenous to the United States, however; many of these are found world wide. As I have traveled around the globe I have found quite a number of these in many places. I have tried to give attention, particularly, to the most commonly used herbs in North America. Because there are over 80 herbs in this section, it does not mean that the person reading this book is required to use all 80 of them. I have listed this many simply as an endeavor to provide a broad based, quality education in herbology such that wherever you go on this continant or to other parts of the world, there may be several herbs that you recognize and may be able to work with. Most herbalists find that they work with a far smaller number of herbs on a consistant basis than are listed.

Dosages

The dosage recomendations provided in this book are safe for *most* **adults**. In fact they should be safe for all people. However, at this point in time not all men are equal! On rare occasions we find that some unique individuals will either not realize enough effect at the suggested dosage level or may conversly discover that a typical dosage is to high for them. **Childrens dosages** may be derived by using a mathematical formula. The adult dosages are based on assuming that the adult is between 125 and 175 lbs. Determine a child's dose by dividing the child's weight by the average adult weight and multipliying the result times the adult dosage. For an example: Assume that you wish to treat a 45lb. child. > 45/150 = .3 .3 x 6 caps = 1.8 caps. You will have to choose to either use 2 caps or one full cap and one cap from which you remove a 1/5 of the herb. You may use the same type logic for infusions, decoctions, and tinctures.

Aloe >

Latin description: Aloe vera also known as Aloe
   barbadensis.
Lesser known variety: Aloe ferox, source for cape aloe.

Parts to use: Leaves. Leaves yield juice, gel, and a dried
   leaf powder.

Chemical constituents: Gel: Acetylated mannon, steroidal
   substances, amino acids, saponins, enzymes. Outer
   leaf: anthraquinone glycosides.

Applications and uses: The gel obtained by filleting the
   leaves is an effective soothing remedy for scrapes and
   especially burns. When applying to burns, it can be
   made more effective by mixing with honey and vitamin
   E oil. The gel also is soothing to the G.I. tract but care
   must be taken to avoid ingesting any of the outer leaf.
   Many commercial preparations are available but most
   are not of much use. The dried powder of the outer
   leaf can be a laxative. The powder made from the aloe
   ferox (called Cape aloe) is used to promote proper
   function of a sluggish colon (short term).

Dosage >
   Gel: apply as needed.
   Capsules: 2 capsules of outer leaf powder once or
      twice daily. Not for long term use.

American Cranesbill > Also Known as: Wild geranium &
   spotted cranesbill.

Latin description: Geranium maculatum.

Parts to use: Rhizome.

Chemical constituents: Natural resin, tannic acid, gallic
   acid.

Applications and uses: Cranesbill powder is fantastic for
   stopping internal hemorrhaging and also external
   bleeding. Some find it useful to make a gargle for sore
   throats and other oral sores. May also be used in cases
   of diarrhea although it wouldn't be my first choice.

Dosage >
   Decoction: 1/2 cup per application until bleeding
      stops. More effective when combined with
      cayenne.

Arnica >

Latin description: Arnica montana.

Parts to use: dried flowers.

Chemical constituents: thymol, arnicin.

Applications and uses: Externally used in salves or oils as an
   antibacterial for treating scrapes, cuts and abrasions.
   Will also relieve painful joints when applied topically. It
   would be helpful to mix wintergreen oil or peppermint
   oil with it to help carry the arnica in deeper.

Dosage >
   External use only unless directed by an experienced
   practitioner.

Astragalus > Also known as: Huang qi and mil-vetch.

Latin description: Astragalus membranacues.

Parts to use: Root.

Chemical constituents: Betaine, choline, glycosides, glucornic Acid, and sucrose.

Applications and uses: Builds and strengthens the immune system. Works well to strengthen the digestive system. Will also defeat long term fatigue as it supports normal adrenal function. Can be useful in ending a debilitating sweat during illness. Strangely enough it may produce a sweat in situations as it is desired. Some practitioners find Astragalus a useful aid in healing chronic ulcers. May also have a mild diuretic effect.

Dosage >
Capsules: 6 "0" capsules daily.
Decoction: 1 root slice every other day in 1 pint water, may be used long term.

Barberry > Also known as: Berberi, wood sour, pepperidge bush.

Latin description: Berberis vulgaris.

Parts to use: Bark, root bark, and berries.

Chemical constituents: Berbamine, berberine, berberrubine, columbamine, hydrastine, jatorrhizine, manganese, oxycanthine, palmatine.

Applications and uses: Externally used in preparations to

kill bacteria. Internally used as a laxative. Will slow rapid heart rate and respiration. Best used as a liver cleanser. Helpful in conditions of enlarged spleen.

Dosage >
Capsules: 2-4 "0" capsules 3x daily max.
Decoction: 1 cup 3x daily before meals.

Bearberry > See Uva Ursi.

Bladderwrack > Also known as: Kelp.

Latin description: Fucusvesiculosus.

Parts to use: Entire plant.

Chemical constituents: Mucilage, mannitol, alginic acid, iodine, potassium and a wide spectrum of trace minerals.

Applications and uses: Has been used to combat obesity. I suspect the benefits in dealing with obesity results from its iodines that support the thyroid gland therefore increasing metabolic function and lowering the bodies ability to store fats. Has also been used in conditions of rheumatism and arthritis. It can be applied externally in compresses or possibly plasters to use on the local inflammation or swelling that is associated with arthritis.

Dosage >
Best used in powder. Capsules: 6 "0" capsules daily.

Black Cohosh > Also known as: Snake root and squaw root.

Latin description: Cimicifuga racemosa.

Parts to use: Dried root and rhizome.

Chemical constituents: Triterpene-glycosides, resin,
   salicylates, oleic acid, palmation acid, phosphorus,
   isoferulic acid, ranunculin, tannin, traces of estrogenic
   substances.

Applications and uses: Primary use is as an antispasmodic.
   Black cohosh is a tremendous remedy in dealing with
   both whooping cough and asthma. Used quite effectively for menstrual cramps and also the spasmodic
   action and muscle tension in rheumatoid arthritis. It has
   salicylates which are antiinflammatory and makes this
   doubly helpful in dealing with arthritis and also in
   respiratory disorders. It is also a mild sedative and will
   work well with other antispasmodics and nervines in
   decreasing pain.

Dosage >
   Capsules: No more than 3 "0" capsules per hour.
       Typical dosage would be 1-3 capsules 3x daily.
   Decoction: Drink 1 cup 3x daily max.

Blessed Thistle > Also known as: Holy thistle, benedicten
   thistle, st. benedict thistle, blessed cardus.

Latin description: Cardus benedictus.

Parts to use: Root, aerial parts and the seeds.

Chemical constituents: Mucilage, essential oil, cincin,
   tannin.

Applications and uses: Primarily used for relactation. It can
   be used to increase the flow of a mother's milk that is

already in full lactation. Less common usage is as a mild diuretic and may be used to induce sweating if that is desired. It may also be used to help regenerate the liver. It is also useful in situations where you have inflammation in the lungs such as bronchitis and pleurisy. Some claim that Blessed Thistle is an appetite stimulant.

CAUTION: If taken in large dosages you have danger of it being an emetic and a possible cause of diarrhea.

Dosage >
  Capsules: 4 "0" capsules 4x daily.
  Infusion: (aerial parts) No more than 1/2 cup every
    two hours.
  Decoction: (Root and seeds) No more than 1/2 cup
    every two hours.

Blue Cohosh > Also known as: Blue ginseng, squaw root,
    papoose root.

  Latin description: Caulophyllum thalictroides.

  Parts to Use: Root and rhizome.

  Chemical constituents: Alkaloids, coulosaponin, inositol,
    iron, magnesium, leontin, nethylcystine, phosphoric acid,
    phosphorus, potassium, silicon, baptifoline, anagyrine,
    laburinine.

  Applications and uses: Primarily used for dysmenorrhea.
    Since it is an antispasmodic it helps with unusual
    menstrual cramps. Also used in stomach cramps in low
    dosages. It can be used with anti-inflammatories in
    arthritis compounds because it relieves muscle spasm
    activities that pull on the joints and makes the inflamma-

tion worse. It has been historically used for some time both in natural human medicine and also in veterinary medicine to drink a tea or make an infusion a few weeks before giving birth. It helps to make the birthing process easier, however, it should be used in this instance with extreme caution. Blue Cohosh should only be used during pregnancy in the last two to three weeks of the pregnancy. It can be beneficial in providing an easier and faster labor but should be administered by an experienced herbal practitioner.

CAUTION: Normally not used during pregnancy, in cases of heart disease, or in cases of high blood pressure.

Dosage >
    Capsules: 4 "0" capsules 3-4x daily max. May be unsafe for some. Would highly recommend starting with a lower dose.
    Decoction: Take 2 ounces 3-4x daily.

Burdock > Also known as: Cocklebur, beggar button, cockle button.

Latin description: Arctium lappa.

Parts to use: Roots, leaves and seeds (mainly the roots).

Chemical Constituents: Fresh Roots: insulin, polyacetylenes, acidic acid, proprionic acid, butyric acid, isovaleric acid, lauric acid, palmitic acid, stearic acid, myristic acid, manganese, sulphur, biotin, tannin. Seeds: arctiin, chlorogenic acid. Leaves: arctiol, fukinone, taraxasterol.

Applications and uses: Blood purifier, tissue purifier. You

use it in mild amounts and not in heavy dosages. It has somewhat of a laxative property, and is a mild diuretic. Burdock root and leaves can be used in internal and external preparations for skin disorders such as psoriasis and eczema. A decoction of the root is restorative to the liver and gallbladder functions and has a mild stimulating effect to the immune system. It has an antimicrobial action which makes it useful in treating skin disorders such as boils, acne, and other skin infections. You would use this primarily with an external plaster. Its antimicrobial property may also be useful internally. It is useful in cases of cysts in the urinary tract. One valuable use for the root especially is in decoctions for eliminating acids in alleviating the symptoms of both osteo arthritis and rheumatoid arthritis. The fresh leaves are quite bitter and can be useful in stimulating purification of the liver. Bone spurs and related calcifications may be removed by drinking up to a quart of the decoction of burdock root daily for 2-3 weeks. Even better results are obtained if you also take 8-14 alfalfa tablets daily while drinking the decoction. **CAUTION**: People who are suffering with hypoglycemia should use with care as burdock can lower blood sugar levels.

Dosage >
Capsules: 4 "0" capsules of root powder 4x daily max.
Decoction: Drink 3 cups twice daily.

Butchers Broom > Also known as: Broom.

Latin description: Ruscus aculeatus.

Parts to use: Seeds and seed top.

Chemical constituents: Hydroxytyramine, alkaloids, ruscogenins.

Applications and uses: Butchers broom has a mild anti-inflammatory action. Primarily used in situations where we have reduced circulation especially in the extremities. It is quite useful in most instances in lowering high blood pressure. In rare instances it can do the reverse, so start out with a low dosage. It works quite well to increase circulation where you have occluded arteries or thrombosis. Caution, don't use for thrombosis unless directed by a physician or other qualified natural practitioner. It is a useful remedy in cases of phlebitis. Because of its ability to increase circulation it is an excellent remedy for preventing the destructive side of diabetes on the circulatory system.

Dosage >
Capsules: Up to 3 "0" capsules 2x daily. It is recommended to start with 1 capsule two times daily and increase until the desired affect is achieved without over dosing.

Catnip > Also known as: Cat Mint.

Latin description: Nepeta cataria.

Parts to use: Aerial.

Chemical constituents: Acidic acid, butyric acid, choline, sitral, inositol, thymol, volatile oils, tannins, PABA, phosphorus, sodium, sulphur, valeric acid, limonene, lifronella, dipentene.

Applications and uses: Catnip works well as a antispasmodic in case of diarrhea and cramping. It works as a mild sedative to help in insomnia. It may be used to calm an upset stomach, and is a tremendous tool in dealing with colic. If you are going to be doing a high enema and you do not want the spastic action in the colon you may use some of the catnip in the enema as a tea and it will prevent this. It helps to stimulate sweating, so it is excellent in dealing with colds and flus. It has been reported to stimulate the appetite and aid in digestion.

Dosage >
Capsules: A maximum of 3 "0" capsules 4x daily.
Infusions: Drink 1 cup 3x daily.

Cat's Claw > Also known as: Una de gato.

Latin Description: Unicaria tomentosa.

Parts to use: Inner bark.

Chemical Constituents: Alkaloids, polyphenols, triterpenes, betasitosterol, stigmasterol, campasterol.

Applications and uses: Antiinflammatory, antiviral. Blocks fluid retention, stimulates immune system. Is an anti-angiogenic herb. Used in crohns disease.

Dosage>
Capsules: 3 caps 3x daily.
Decoction: 3 cups daily.

Cayenne > Also known as: Bird pepper.

Latin description: Capsicum frutescens.

Parts to use: Pods.

Chemical Constituents: Capsaicin, apsaicine, carotenoids, flavonoids, volatile oils, capsacutin, capsathine, PABA, capsico.

Applications and uses: Cayenne is useful in lowering blood pressure. It should only be taken short term. It is an excellent gargle for sore throat and oral ulcers. It allays the pain as well as purifying and cleansing. It is antibacterial. Cayenne is a tremendous remedy for stopping bleeding both internally and externally. It is indicated in use for arthritis internally and externally. If you do not have access to medical attention and some one is having a heart attack, several capsules orally may be quite beneficial towards keeping the heart beating and regulating the beat. Cayenne will also stay off and avert the heart attack temporarily. It can be used internally and externally for pleurisy. It is also a systemic stimulant. It is not a neurological stimulant or a nervous system stimulant like many of the other stimulants that we know of like caffeine, etc. Used on a short term basis it can be good for increasing vitality overall. Cayenne should be understood to be a natural medicine and not a long term food product. Many people use it as a dietary mainstay as far as a seasoning or a flavoring and that should probably not be done. There is controversy surrounding cayenne as part of the diet. Although it does appear that cayenne can be an irritant to the digestive system, that seems to only be where it is cooked and not taken simply as a dried and ground product.

Chaparral > Also known as: Creosote bush.

Latin description: Larrea divaricata.

Parts to use: Leaves.

Chemical constituents: Sodium, sulphur, nordihydroquaiaretic acid.

Applications and uses: Chaparral is a free radical scavenger and a cancer fighter. When mixed with Goldenseal, Chaparral helps to draw toxic chemicals and even street drugs out of the cells and suspends them in the blood. These make both a good cellular and tissue cleanse. You must start slowly as rapid detoxification can be detrimental. It helps to improve liver function. It is a good blood purifier. It has an antiviral, antibacterial, antiparasitic action. It is very cleansing to the urinary system. If you are a person who has had a lot of chemotherapy or other type of drug therapies it may cause nausea or other types of side effects as it releases those substances from the tissues into the blood stream. **CAUTION: Long term usage may cause liver complication.**

Dosage >
Capsules: 3-6 "0" capsules 3x daily.
Infusion: 1 cup 3x daily.

Chaste Tree Berry > Also known as: Chaste berry, monks pepper.

Latin description: Vitex agnus castus.

Parts to use: fruit or berry.

Chemical constituents: Volatile oils, castine, flavonoids, glycosides.

Applications and uses: Primarily used in dealing with disorders of the female reproductive organs. It is of great benefit in dealing with both PMS and menopause. It aids in regulating the estrogen balance in the body. It is quite useful in dissolving fibroid tumors. Chaste tree berries are also good for reestablishing the normal cycle of ovulation and menstruation if it has been disrupted by contraceptives or such. It increases the production of Luteinizing hormone, and the secretion of Prolactin. This of course would be corollary with the stimulation of lactation. It is very beneficial in instances where menstruation is either too frequent, prolonged, or when the flow is heavier than normal.

Dosage >
    Not recommended for decoctions.
    Capsules: 2 "0" capsules 3x daily for most disorders.
    More may be used for helping with lactation.
    Tincture: 9 drops 3x daily.

Chickweed >

Latin description: Stellaria Media.

Parts to use: Aerial.

Chemical constituents: saponins, mucilage, choline, copper, phosphorus, PABA, biotin, traces of several vitamins.

Applications and uses: Used in external applications for skin diseases such as dermatitis, eczema, and psoriasis.

We also use it in treating skin diseases by including it in various oils and in tinctures externally. Internally we use this in treating bronchial problems such as coughs, bronchitis. Chickweed is effective in reducing the mucous in the lungs and acts as an expectorant to bring the mucous up. It has been used in past times in rheumatism and works on that particular condition as an anti inflammatory.

Dosage >
Capsules: 4 "0" capsules 3x daily.
Infusion: Drink 1 cup 3x daily. It is difficult to over dose on this since many people use this as a salad vegetable.

Chamomile > Also known as: Ground apple, Roman chamomile.

Latin description: Anthemis nobilis.

Parts to use: Aerial.

Chemical constituents: salicylates, cyanogenic glycosides, follicle oil, flavonoids including rutin, valerinic acid, anthene acid, anthesterol, apigenin, chanazulene, tannic acid, tiglic acid.

Applications and uses: Chamomile has a very mild nervine and aids in dealing with insomnia. It is an old remedy for headaches. It has been used in the treatment of rheumatism and arthritis, as it does have a bit of an antiinflammatory affect. Chamomile is used as an antiemetic. It is used as an eye wash in conjunctivitis. It can be used in preparations in treating bronchial catarrh such as bronchitis, asthma, and hay fever. Chamomile tea was used in earlier times for whooping cough because of its ability to clear out matter in the lungs but also because of its antispasmodic action. There is also an antifungal property in chamomile which makes it a good wash externally and also internally in dealing with thrush. You can also make an essential oil and use it topically for thrush. It has an antibacterial agent in it that works quite well in treating staph infections.

Dosage >
Capsules: Up to 8 capsules 3x daily max.
Infusion: Drink 1 cup 3x daily.

Comfrey > Also known as: Knit bone, bruise wart.

Latin description: Cymphytum officinale.

Parts to use: Roots, leaves.

Chemical constituents: mucilage, allantioim, tannins, essential oils, gum, pyrrolizioline, alkaloids, beta-sitosterol, steroidal saponins, triterpenoids, Vit. B-12, phosphorus, potassium.

Applications and uses: Comfrey makes a tremendous poultice because it has allanton, which causes cell proliferation.* It helps cause rapid growth of the tissues, especially connective tissues, bone, cartilage as some of those areas are hard to heal. Comfrey has been called the vegetable DMSO. It absorbs and is easily transported through skin, tissues, and cell membranes. It tends to break down red blood cells, which is probably how it got its name as bruise wart. Comfrey leaf is good as a poultice to alleviate bruises and dissolve and dispel them rapidly. Comfrey can also be used in poultices or compresses for varicose veins. It is tremendous in healing and drawing inflammation, infections, and infected matter out of burns. For internal use, we use it with caution though it is useful in treating bronchitis and other lower respiratory problems. Internally as an infusion it can be useful in loosening mucous in sinuses when they are impacted. It has been a traditional remedy in ulcers. It has a substance that depresses the secretion of a Prostaglandin which is related to inflammatory problems in the stomach or in the GI tract. There has been a caution with internal usage because research has correlated heavy internal use with liver cancer. Consequently we would place a caution with Comfrey regarding excessive internal consumption.

Dosage >
Capsules: 5-10 "0" capsules up to 3x daily.
Infusion: Drink 1 cup 3x daily.
*Caution: Avoid internal use with cancer patients or those with increased risk.

Couch Grass > Also known as: Witch grass, dog grass, twitch grass, quick grass, and most commonly quack grass.

Latin description: Adropyron retens.

Parts to use: Rhizome.

Chemical constituents: Mannitol, vanillin glycoside, saponin, mucilage, potassium silica, iron, volatile oil, triticin, inositol.

Applications and uses: The volatile oil in it makes it useful as a broad spectrum antibiotic. It is quite useful in treating urinary tract infections. Some herbalists have had good success in treating both urinary stones and also the inflammation of the prostate gland using couch grass.

Dosage >
Decoction: 1-3 cups daily.

Cleavers > Also known as: Goose grass, sticky grass.

Latin description: Galium aparine.

Parts to use: Aerial.

Chemical constituents: Tannins, citric acid, coumarins, glycosides.

Applications and uses: Is useful in cleansing the lymphatic system. Can be useful in some instances to lower blood pressure which may be due to the fact that it is an excellent diuretic. It is reliable in cleansing the urinary tract and an excellent item to use in preparations to treat urinary infections. Also useful in helping to lower the body temperature in fevers. Externally it can be used both to treat dandruff and some naturalists have discovered that they can make a natural body deodorant from the infusion.

Dosage >
Capsules: 3 "0" capsules 3x daily.
Infusion: 1 cup 3x daily.
　　　Usage should be restricted to short term, no longer than four or five days for internal use.

Cramp Bark > Also known as: High bush cranberry, snowball bush, guelder rose.

Latin description: Viburnum opulus.

Parts to use: Bark.

Chemical constituents: Valeric acid, salicosides, tannin, viburnin.

Applications and uses: Internally-it is used as a muscle relaxant. It is of great benefit in easing excessive cramping associated with menstruation. It can be used during pregnancy with caution to prevent miscarriage. It is also used with supervision for heart palpitation or irregular heart rates.
CAUTION: Do not eat the berries!

Dosage >
Capsules: 4-9 "0" capsules 3x daily.
Decoction: 1 cup 3x daily.

Dandelion > Also known as: Lions teeth.

Latin description: Taraxacum officinale.

Parts to use: Flowers, leaves, and roots.

Chemical constituents: Root- bitter glycosides, carotenoids, terpenoids, insulin, pectin, choline, phenolic acid, potassium. Leaves-lutein, biolaxanthin, carotenoids, potassium, iron, Vit-A content in these leaves is even higher than in carrots.

Applications and uses: The leaves are a liver tonic and

33

since they are bitter they may also be a digestive tonic. They are also quite effective as a diuretic, hence its French slang term; Pee- in- the- bed. The root is also a tremendous liver tonic. We use it extensively in purging and cleansing the liver. It strengthens the flow of the bile. It also has a mild diuretic effect.

Dosage >
Capsules: Leaves- 5 "0" capsules 3x daily.
Capsules: Root - 4 "0" capsules 3x daily.
Decoction: Root - 1 cup 3x daily.
Infusion: Leaves - 1 cup 4x daily.

Echinacea > Also known as: Snake root, Missouri snake root, black samson, purple cone flower.

Latin description: Echinacea angustifolia or echinacea purpurea. There are several varieties. Preference would be given to the Echinacea Angustifolia because it is more potent and more powerful in its effects.

Parts to use: Dried root and rhizome.

Chemical constituents: Arabinose, betaine, echinacn, fatty acids, galactose, glucose, glucuronic acid, inulin, inuloid, humulene, caryophylene, glycoside, polysaccharides, polyacetylenes, sobutylalklamines, resins, sesquiterpne.

Applications and uses: Echinacea is a very powerful immune system stimulator. It stimulates production of white blood cells for fighting infection. The polysaccharides have strong antiviral properties. It is an effective natural antibiotic. The external use would be as a poultice for boils, bites, abscesses, and other infections. It is useful where you have swollen lymph

34

nodes or glands. The main use for this herb though, would be to boost the immune system and for fighting infections. You may also use a decoction of the root when you have a purulent or external infection and wash it with this such as an abscess or ulcer. It would be very purifying and cleansing as a topical antibiotic application.

Dosage >
Capsules: 2-8 "0" capsules 3x daily.
Decoction: Drink 1 cup 4x daily.
Alcohol tinctures of Echinacea are not recommended because they destroy the polysaccharides that stimulate the immune system so you would not get the immune response from this as you would from the decoction or the infusion.

Elecampane > Also known as: Elfdoc, wild sunflower, yellow star wart.

Latin description: Inula helenium.

Parts to use: Root and rhizome.

Chemical constituents: Alantolactone, isoalantalactone, azulne, inulin, sterols, resins, mucilage.

Applications and uses: In the earlier history of the United States medical practitioners used Elecampane as a specific treatment for tuberculosis. It is an excellent expectorant. Elecampane works well for bronchitis, bronchial infections, and pulmonary infections. It can be used in conjunction with other herbs in treating asthma. It can be used to expel intestinal parasites. Because it is quite bitter it can be quite beneficial as a liver tonic, causing the liver to produce an increased flow of bile. Externally it is good to apply on scabies and herpes lesions. Internally it also can regulate dysmenorrhea.

Dosage >
Capsules: up to 3 "0" capsules 3x daily.
Decoction: 2 cups daily.
Wash: use externally for skin diseases.

Ephedra-Chinese > Also known as: Brigham tea, ma huang.

Latin description: Ephedra sinica.

Parts to use: Aerial, primarily the more tender stems.

Chemical constituents: Ephedrine, norephedrine, methyl ephedrine, pseudoephedrine tannins, saponin, flavone, essential oil.

Applications and uses: Ephedra contains an effective antihistamine. It has some useful properties as a decongestant. It is particularly useful in asthma and hayfever. It has been used to treat high blood pressure in low doses. The volatile oils inhibit viruses and can be used when you feel that you are catching a cold or a flu bug in the early stages to knock it out before it becomes a full blown illness. It can be used in cases of whooping cough. Also in cases where you have an uncontrolled sweat and fever this will help to decrease that.
CAUTION: Should not be taken by people who are on prescription antidepressants. It should also be avoided in cases of glaucoma, hyperthyroidism, coronary thrombosis, severe prostate enlargement, and in cases of severe hypertension. It should be used with

care in any application.

Dosage>
Capsules: 2 "0" capsules 2x daily (possibly 3x daily).
Infusion: Drink 1/4 cup 3x daily.

Eucalyptus > Also known as: Blue gum.

Latin description: Eucalyptus globulus.

Parts to use: Leaves.

Chemical constituents: Oil, cineole, pinenes, sesquiterpene
alcohol, aromadendrene, cuminaldehyde.

Applications and uses: The oil is an antiseptic and can be
used externally on the skin. The antiseptic oil is also
very volatile and can be used in steam inhalations and
will kill germs as it is absorbed into the lungs. It can
also be used in very low dosages in cough syrups. It
has a tremendous toxic effect on things like fleas or lice.

Dosage >
Generally not recommended for oral use, however,
several drops may be used in cough syrups.

Evening Primrose > Also known as: Primrose. Latin
description: Oenothera lanarkiana.

Parts to use: Oil, gotten from both the plant and seeds.

Chemical constituents: Gama-linolenic acid (also known as
GLA), linoleic acid.

Applications and uses: Primrose aids in restoring livers

that have been damaged by alcohol or other chemical exposures. It has been proven to be valuable in multiple sclerosis in preventing demyelinization. It is effective in treating rheumatoid arthritis because of the GLA. GLA is also found in Flaxseed. One would be careful to make certain that the oil extraction process is a cold extraction otherwise the GLA will have been changed to another chemical form which would be carcinogenic. Evening Primrose has clinical studies associated showing significant alleviation of ADD (Attention Deficit Disorder). It is very effective in dealing with PMS.

CAUTION: It is not recommended for use in conditions of epilepsy. It is possible to cause skin sensitivities but not very likely.

Dosage >

The oil can be taken in drops and is typically sold commercially in gelatin caps that contain animal products, and we don't recommend using the gelatin caps. You can prick a hole in the gelatin cap and squirt the oil out of it and take the oil this way. Commercially prepared oils vary in potency; take as directed on the bottle or you can make your own oil and take possibly 20-35 drops of the oil per day. If purchased in International Units take up to 2600IU daily.

Eye Bright >

Latin Description: Euphrasia officinalis.

Parts to use: Aerial.

Chemical constituents: glycosides, saponins, tannins, resin, volatile oil.

Applications and uses: Use eye bright to make an excellent
eye wash. It can be applied externally as a compress
or a wash to irritated or infected eyes. Eye bright can
be combined with Goldenseal, Fennel, and or Red
Sumac berries for Pink Eye or Conjunctivitis. It can be
taken internally for weak eyes. It has been reported to
be effective in early stages of cataracts. Eye bright is
also an astringent and can be used as such in an external
wash. It effects the liver and blood and can be used to
detoxify both. An infusion is effective in dealing with
nasal congestion that comes with hayfever and colds or
may also be used as a mouth wash for irritations of the
mucous membranes.

Dosage >
Capsules: 4 "0" capsules up to 4x daily.
Infusion: 1 cup 4x daily.

Fenugreek > Also known as: Greek seed, bird foot.

Latin description: Trigonella foenum-graecum.

Parts to use: Seeds.

Chemical constituents: Trigonelline, choline, gentianine,
biotin, inositol, lecethin, mucilage, diosgenin, flavonoids,
PABA, trimethylamine.

Applications and uses: Fenugreek is a tremendous decongestant. It is good for clearing congested sinuses.
Some people use it with hot flashes due to menopause.
You will find that it is of great benefit in increasing
lactation for nursing mothers. It is also used as a

flavoring or spice. Use fenugreek for making poultices for boils or other infected external sores. Because it does have a uterine stimulant it should not be used during pregnancy except with caution.

Dosage >
Capsules: up to 5 "0" capsules 3x daily. The herb is usually considered to bitter to be used in an infusion.

Feverfew >

Latin description: Tanacetum parthenium.

Parts to use: Dried flowers, leaves, and more tender stems.

Chemical constituents: Borneol, camphor, arthenolide, pyrethrins, santamarin, terpene, volatile oil, tannins.

Applications and uses: For migraine headaches, rheumatoid and osteo arthritis. It has an excellent antiinflammatory mechanism different than most antiinflammatories and it works well toward relieving the inflammation and pain from arthritis. It can also be used in conjunction with asthma as it prevents spasms in the smaller blood vessels.
CAUTION: Some people notice an increase in oral ulcers with regular use though it is unlikely.

Dosage >
Capsules: up to 3 "0" capsules 3x daily, however, that is a rather elevated dosage and should be used for only a short time at that dosage. It would be better to drop down to 1 capsule 3x daily after one week of using.
Infusion: 1 cup 2x daily.

Garlic >

Latin description: Allium aativu.

Parts to use: Bulb.

Chemical constituents: Volatile oils, allicin, alliin, ajoene, phosphorus, magnesium, germanium, allyldisulfides, selenium, phytoncides.

Applications and uses: Antibiotic. It is a mild expectorant. It is useful in counteracting high blood pressure. In larger dosages it can be useful as an anti-coagulant. Garlic is a recognized remedy against both high cholesterol and arterial plaque. It also is effective in reducing high blood sugar in diabetes. Internally the use of garlic is effective in reducing the incidence of stroke. Garlic can be used against diarrhea, TB, diptheria, typhoid, hepatitis and other types of infectious diseases. The antifungal component in garlic is very effective against candida by ingesting supplemental forms. The antifungal properties are also quite useful in expelling intestinal parasites, also cleaning up athletes foot. Externally it can be used in liquid form on acne and it works very well as a purative on external sores and infections. It can be used in an oil form or liquid form as an excellent remedy for ear aches and infection, placing it directly in the ear canal. There is much research that indicates that garlic is quite positive in increasing the immune system response. Research has also shown that it actually works actively against cancer. Cold aged extracts are proven to be significantly more effective than other types of garlic.

Dosage >
>   Capsules: 2 or more "0" capsules of the powder may
    be taken daily on a long term bases. If you are
    taking a therapeutic dose for short term you may
    take 8-10 capsules daily.
>   Oil: 4-5 drops as for an ear problem, into the ear
    canal.

Ginkgo > Also known as: Maiden hair tree.

Latin description: Ginkgo biloba.

Parts to use: Leaves and seeds, though the use of the
    seeds is uncommon.

Chemical constituents: Leaves-ginkgolides, heterosids,
    bioflavones, sitosterol, lactones, anthocyanin.
    Seeds- bioflavones, fatty acids.

Applications and uses: Primarily to increase brain function.
    It increases peripheral circulation. It increases the
    capacity of the blood to carry oxygen. It also increases
    blood flow to the peripheral areas such as the brain and
    the extremities. Indicated in usage with memory loss,
    Alzhiemers disease. It can be quite useful with irregular
    heart beat or arrythmia. Externally the leaves can be
    used in poultices or compresses for hemorrhoids or
    varicose veins. I find it particularly useful in reducing
    arterial plaque. It is a relatively safe herb and advanced
    usage is not considered dangerous, although higher or
    therapeutic dosages should be reached gradually and
    discontinued gradually as well. The seeds have an anti-
    bacterial and antifungal action and are typically used
    externally but can also be used internally. With the
    seeds we are much more cautious for internal use and

would probably not use more than 3 seeds per day and would not use it long term.

Dosage >
   Capsules: 3 "0" capsules 2-3x daily.
   Infusion: 1 cup 2x daily.

Goldenrod >

Latin description: Solidago virgaurea.

Parts to use: Aerial.

Chemical constituents: Flavonoids, essential oil, tannins.

Applications and uses: Goldenrod is useful in clearing gravel from the urinary tract and is also effective in cleansing the urinary tract in the case of urinary tract infections. It helps to eliminate toxins in the kidneys and tissues. Therefore it may also be useful in an infusion for arthritis. You may find Goldenrod very useful in clearing mucous in upper airways, therefore it is indicated in both lower and upper respiratory infections. It has been proven useful in bronchitis, pneumonia, pleurisy, etc. Typically Goldenrod is not a stand alone herb, but may be combined with Mullien or other herbs that are useful in those parts of the body.

Dosage >
   Capsules: up to 3 "0" capsules 2-3 times daily.
   Infusion: up to 3 cups daily.

Goldenseal > Also known as: Yellow root, Indian turmeric.

Latin description: Hydrastis canadensis.

Parts to use: Root and rhizome.

Chemical constituents: Hydrastine, berberine, candine, choline, chologenic acid, inositol, lignin, PABA, volatile oil, resin.

Applications and uses: Goldenseal is a tremendous remedy against inflammations in the mucous membranes. Goldenseal is valuable in dealing with conditions in the mouth such as infections and inflammations of the gums and other oral tissues. You will find it useful in dealing with ulcers elsewhere in the gastrointestinal tract. It has an antiyeast and antifungal effects and is excellent as a douche in dealing with thrush or yeast infections vaginally. Make it into a tea and use as a compress on eyes, or drops of infusion to be placed directly into the eye. Also may be used as a poultice on skin eruptions and infections. Some people use it as a remedy for morning sickness, but because of the berberine, which is a uterine stimulator, it is not indicated during pregnancy. Goldenseal also is indicated to use with ring worm and other skin eruptions and infections. It very strongly stimulates the liver into producing elevated quantities of bile so is a good liver purgative. It has a very effective antibacterial, antiviral, and anti-fungal properties and can be used as antibiotic both internally and externally. Tinctures and other preparations may be used in dealing with funguses under fingernails, toe nails, and also on the skin itself. Goldenseal is quite useful in dealing with cases of food poisoning as it destroys both the microorganism that has gotten into the gastrointestinal tract and also whatever toxins that they are releasing into the system. It has a mild antiinflammatory effect. Is also used as a digestive tonic. Because of its uterine contracting possibilities it would be indicated in use where there is excessive uterine bleeding, perhaps postpartum.   Short term use is indicated in diabetes because of its potentiating of insulin. It potentiates the use of insulin. Goldenseal is also indicated for use in prostate inflammation. **CAUTION:** Do not use during pregnancy. Do not use for more than 10 days consecutively without giving several weeks off of it in between, as there is a property that tends to build up in the liver and causes the liver to become toxic over long term use.

Dosage >
    Capsules: up to 4 "0" capsules 4x daily for only 10
        days and then off for 2 weeks.
    Infusion: 1 cup up to 4x daily for one week.

Gotu Kola > Also known as: Indian penny wart.

Latin description: Hydrocotyle asiatica.

Parts to use: Aerial.

Chemical constituents: Heteroside, asiaticoside, catechol, epicatechol, glycosides, resins, tannins, volatile oils, traces of theobromine.

Applications and uses: It has typically been used for Tuberculosis and leprosy, because it is a blood tonic and blood purifier. We know that the life is in the blood. It is an excellent remedy against mental disorders such as depression. Gotu kola can be used to combat high blood pressure and congestive heart failure. In low doses it is effective with insomnia. Gotu kola can be used as a mild diuretic. It helps regulate both liver and heart function, but should be used in fairly low doses and not used over very long terms. When combined with feverfew it is an excellent remedy for migraines. Also in combination with ginkgo it is excellent in increasing alertness & memory capacity.

Dosage >
    Capsules: 1-3 "0" capsules 2x daily. Large or long term doses are not recommended and should be used with caution.
    Infusion: 1/2 cup 2x daily.

Gravel Root > Also known as: Queen of the meadow, gravel weed, and joe-pye weed.

Latin description: Eupatorium purpureum.

Parts to use: Roots and rhizome.

Chemical constituents: Flavonoids, volatile oil, resin, tannins, sesquiterpene, lactones.

Applications and uses: A decoction of the root is drunk for a variety of complaints. Included are pelvic inflammations, prostate inflammations, urinary infections, kidney stones. It has a diuretic effect which causes the purging of uric acid which of course would give it excellent consideration in gout, rheumatism, and arthritis. Also it is used to relieve severe menstrual cramping and pain.

Dosage >
    Capsules: 4 "0" capsules 3x daily.
    Decoction: 1-2 cups daily.

Hawthorn > Also known as: White thorn, may blossom.

Latin description: Crategus oxyacantha.

Parts to use: Flowers and berries.

Chemical constituents: choline, citric acid, cratagolic acid, flavonoids, flavonoid glycosides, saponins, inositol, glavone, procyanidines, trimethylamine, tannins.

Applications and uses: The berries are a tremendous answer to high blood pressure, used beautifully to dilate coronary and peripheral arteries. The berries can be used in compounds where you are dealing with rapid heart beat. The compounds in the berries help the heart to have both a stronger and a more effective contractions as to pump more blood for the effort. Hawthorn can be utilized in conditions of low blood pressure as well. It is excellent in respect to angina and arrythmia. The flowers are useful in dealing with persons who have very weak hearts relative to post heart attack or old age. There are some indications that it may lower cholesterol. In some situations they are useful in dealing with abdominal pain and diarrhea. You may also use the decoction of the berries in cases of insomnia.

Dosage >
    Capsules: 1-4 "0" capsules 3x daily. Most individu-
    als can do quite well with 1 capsule 3x daily.
    The elevated dose should be done with caution.
    Decoction: Berries: 1/2 cup 3x daily.

Horehound >

Latin Description: Marrubium vulgare.

Parts to use: Tops.

Chemical constituents: Marrubin, volatile oils, resins, tannins.

Applications and uses: Horehound is typically made into syrups and tinctures for colds, asthma, and cough. It is sometimes used in cough drops. It tends to work on soothing and deadening some of the itch that causes the cough. When taken internally it sometimes has a positive effect on reducing flatulence. Horehound is known to be a fairly good expectorant. Horehound can be used with relatively positive effect on lowering blood pressure as it helps to dilate blood vessels and increase peripheral circulation.
CAUTION: It is recommended to be cognizant of what your blood pressure is before starting to use this herb as it may tend to lower it.

Dosage >
Capsules: up to 6 "0" capsules daily.
Infusion: 1-2 cups daily.

Hops >

Latin description: Humulus lupulus.

Parts to use: Flowers from the female plant (Strobiles).

Chemical constituents: Volatile oils, valerianic acid, estrogenic substances, tannins, flavonoids, astralagin, quercitrin, rutin, lumulone, lupulone, linalool, citral, linionene, serolidol, humulene, myrcene, B-cryophyllene, farnescene, lupulin, lupulinic acid, picric acid.

48

Applications and uses: Hops has designations as one of the plants which we call a nervine herb. Its use is for pain, stress, insomnia. A cup of hops tea can be effective in counteracting nervous tension, stomach cramps, also very useful in extreme menstrual cramps. Hops contain antispasmodic and nervines and also because of its estrogenic substances it can help to regulate the menstrual cycle. Since you usually take it as an infusion, it enters the blood stream very rapidly and can give you symptomatic relief very quickly. It can be used either internally as a drink for insomnia, or as in ancient times the people would take the flowers and put them inside of a specific pillow that they would use during periods of insomnia and the evaporation of the volatile oils from the crushing of the plant would have an effect through the olfactory glands and eventually cause sleep due to the sedative effect. It can be a very effective herb in dealing with a spastic colon and disorders such as colitis. I like to use it in preparations when I am dealing with menopause.

CAUTION: In case of mental disease such as depression.

Dosage >
Capsules: 4-6 capsules 3 times daily.
Infusion: 1-2 cups 3 times daily.

Horsetail >

Latin description: Equisetum arvense.

Parts to use: Upper stems.

Chemical constituents: Equisitine, fatty acids, aconitic acid, traces of nicotine.

Applications and uses: It can be beneficial in an individual whose blood is too thin. Also if you have excessive postpartum bleeding or an abnormal menses horsetail is indicated for use. It is high in silica so it is good in compounds for skin conditions. Some of the old herbalists use it to lower fevers. Horsetail has a diuretic effect and can also be used in the application of cleansing the lymphatic system. Horsetail can also be used in an herbal compound of tincture for people who are quitting the smoking habit and have withdrawal symptoms. You would not want to use this long term though on internal applications. Because of its high silica content, people who are having problems with their hair being brittle and excessively dry and also for finger nails and toe nails being easily cracked and broken can benefit from internal use of horsetail.

Dosage >
Capsules: 3 "0" capsules 4x daily max.
Infusion: Maximum of 2 cups daily.

Hydrangea >

Latin Description: Hydrangea arborescens.

Parts to use: Root.

Chemical constituents: Hydrangin, saponin, resin, volatile oil.

Applications and uses: Hydrangea is used when dealing with prostate inflammation and moving and dissolving urinary stones. It can also facilitate the prevention of urinary stones and it has a mild diuretic effect.

Dosage >

> Capsules: up to 9 "0" capsules daily. Typical dosage
> would be short term for 4-6 days. For preventative
> measures use 1-2 caps daily for long term use.
> Decoction: 3 cups daily.

Hyssop >

Latin Description: Hyssopus officinalis.

Parts to use: Aerial, and primarily when it is in bloom.

Chemical constituents: pinocamphone, pinocamphone,
camphene, terpinene, glycosides, tannins, flavonoids,
inoslic acid, oleonolic acid, marrubiin, resins.

Applications and uses: Hyssop is an excellent expectorant.
It is beneficial in treating lower respiratory conditions
such as bronchitis and pneumonia. Hyssop is an herb
that we call diaphoretic which means that it causes a
sweat. You can make an infusion and use it in external
applications for cleansing wounds and for disinfecting
the sick room since it is a good antiseptic. Internally,
hyssop may be good for treating cold sores and canker
sores combined with grape juice as a preventative and
also shortening the duration of the condition.

Dosage >

> Capsules: 2 "0" capsules 4x daily for short term. For
> long term or preventative in dealing with herpes
> simplex viruses take up to 2 capsules daily. We
> typically want to use small dosages of hyssop and
> not to do it for long term uses unless absolutely
> necessary.
> Infusion: 1-1 1/2 cups per daily.

Irish Moss > Also known as: Carragheen.

Latin description: Chondrus crispus.

Parts to use: Fronds or basically the entire plant.

Chemical constituents: polysaccharides, carrageenan, tannins, sodium, sulphur, iodine, bromine, iron, amino acids, sodium.

Applications and uses: It is used sometimes in dietary uses as a gel or a thickening agent. In medical uses it forms a gel or viscous solution internally which coats the gastrointestinal tract which makes it an excellent applications for ulcers. It also seems to inhibit the release or formation of stomach acids which is also somewhat healing for gastric or duodenal ulcers. Irish moss can sometimes be added to the regimen when you are trying to purge gastrointestinal parasites as it, like Slippery Elm, makes the tract very slippery and causes the parasites to pass very easily.

Dosage >
Capsules: up to 16 "0" capsules daily. It is not recommended for long term use as it can decrease the stomach acid and interfere with digestion.
Infusion: It can be simmered with water into a gel and take up to 1 tablespoon in between meals. Irish moss can also be used to gel things when making lotions or creams.

Juniper >

Latin Description: Juniperus communis.

Parts to use: Dried berries.

Chemical constituents: Volatile oils such as pinene, myrcene, sabinene, linonene, terpinene, camphene, thujoene, cadinene, flavones, resins, tannins.

Applications and uses: They are powerful as a diuretic. They stimulate the pancreas. The berries in a decoction is excellent in cleansing the urinary tract. Juniper is quite useful in urinary infections and cystitis. Because of its potent diuretic effect it is very useful in purging various acid crystals from the system and makes it quite beneficial in cases of gout, rheumatism, and arthritis. A decoction makes an excellent antiseptic wash and may be used in instances of vaginal infections, either bacterial or yeast infections. In ancient times the decoctions were used as an antiseptic spray.
CAUTION: Do not use Juniper berries in long term applications. Do not use the larger dosages except in very short term use. Do not use on individuals that have weakened kidneys.

Dosage >
Capsules: 1-2 "0" capsules 4 times daily.
Decoction: Drink 1 cup 2x daily.

Lavender >

Latin description: Lavendula Officionalis.

Parts to use: Flowers; dry.

Chemical constituents: Volatile oils, linabol, linalyl, terpinol, cineole, lavendulyl acetate pinene, limonene coumarins, flavonoids, and camphor.

Applications and uses: Topically used to allay pain on neuralgia and etc. by rubbing on skin. Can be added to massage oils as it will aid in relieving muscle spasms. Excellent as a topical oil to apply to wounds to promote healing. Will disinfect and cleanse thus preventing infection.

Dosage >
Not recommended for internal use unless directed by a professional natural practitioner.

Licorice >

Latin description: Glycyrrhiza glabra.

Parts to use: Root.

Chemical constituents: Flavonoids, Iso flavonoids, sterols, coumarins, amines, Glycyrrhizin.

Applications and uses: Licorice contains natural sterols which can act with steroidal properties. This makes it valuable in cases of arthritis and rheumatism. Helps to buffer when blending herbs with opposing properties. Licorice can be valuable in alleviating the severity of allergic reactions when taken orally.

Dosage>
Capsules: 4 caps 4x daily.
Decoction: 1 cup 4x daily.

Lobelia > Also known as: Indian tobacco.

Latin description: Lobelia inflata.

Parts to use: Aerial.

Chemical constituents: Lobeline, isolobinine, lobelanidine, lobinaline, glycosides, volatile oil, chelidonic acid, selenium, sulphur.

Applications and uses: Lobelia falls into the category of nervines. It is a powerful antispasmodic. It is quite useful in treating asthma and epilepsy. We use it as a potentiator in many other herbal compounds. Lobelia can be included in compounds when helping smokers to kick the habit as it contains substances that help to quell "the urge". Externally it makes an excel lent infusion for use in compresses on muscle sprains, bruises, etc. It was used by old time herbalists for treating epilepsy and lock jaw associated with tetanus. It is also good in lowering long term fevers associated with diseases such as meningitis, pneumonia, and internal infections. **CAUTION:** We are very careful in using Lobelia in large doses as it is an emetic. If taken in too large of or too frequent of a dose the antispasmodic properties could cause the voluntary muscles of the heart and respiration to cease to function which could end in death.

Dosage >
Capsules: 1-2 "0" capsules max. per dosage and per occasion.
Infusion: Take no more than 1 tablespoon at one time. Sip as needed. It is not to be taken on a regular bases.

Marshmallow Root >

Latin description: Althea officinalis.

Parts to use: Root, infrequently leaves.

Chemical constituents: Mucilage which is much higher in the root than the leaves, asparagin, tannin.

Applications and uses: Marshmallow contains a mild expectorant and is used in treating coughs in herbal cough compounds. We use it in the urinary tract any time that we have a urinary tract inflammation or infection. We use it because of its mucilage content to help in moving urinary gravel or stones. It can also be used with Irish Moss or Slippery Elm in conjunction with other herbs for healing of ulcers stomach or GI tract.

Dosage >
   Capsules: 4 "0" capsules 3x daily or more. It is one
      of the few things that you can use freely.
   Decoction: 1 cup 3x daily.

Milk Thistle >

Latin description: Carduus marianus.

Parts to use: Seeds.

Chemical constituents: Silymarin, it acts not only as a flavonoid but as an antioxidant.

Applications and uses: Primarily used in correcting liver conditions. It is an excellent herb in dealing with hepatitis or the recovery. Milk thistle has tremendous regenerating potential relative to the liver. It is helpful in regenerating and stimulating production of new liver cells because of damage either from environmental causes, alcoholism, or chemical exposure. Milk thistle also helps to purify the liver. In many cases, but not all, where food allergies and also environmental allergies are present, this herb would be indicated because in many cases the symptoms in allergies are due to the damage or reduced function of the liver.

Dosage >
> Capsules: A short term therapeutic dose would be 4 "0" capsules 4x daily. A long term maintenance dose would be 1 "0" capsules 4x daily. That should eventually be reduced to 2 capsules daily after 2 months.
> Decoction: Short term: would be 4 cups per day. Long term: would be 1 cup daily.

Motherwort > Also known as: Roman mother wort, lions tail.

Latin description: Leonurus cardiaca.

Parts to use:

Chemical constituents: glycosides, volatile oil, tannins, stachydrine, leonurinine.

Applications and uses: Motherwort can be useful in reducing high blood pressure. It is also useful in rapid and irregular heart beat also heart palpitations. Its primary use is for dealing with irregular menstruation. I have found it to be of great benefit in dealing with the emotional instability of menopause. Motherwort is also an effective uterine stimulator. It can be used in conjunction with other similar herbs for inducing labor, which should only be done under the supervision of an experienced practitioner. Motherwort is quite useful

in reducing post partum bleeding or hemorrhaging. It causes the uterus to clamp down and thus stops the bleeding. It is equally as effective as Ergotamine in causing uterine contractions.
CAUTION: Do not use during pregnancy.

Dosage >
Capsules: Take 4-6 "0" capsules 4x daily.
Infusion: Drink 3 cups daily.

Mullein > Also known as: Aaron's rod, Indian tobacco.

Latin description: Verbascum thapsus.

Parts to use: Leaves, flowers.

Chemical constituents: Saponins, mucilage, aucubin, choline, heseridin, volatile oil, flavonoids, PABA.

Applications and uses: Flowers: can be infused in oil and that oil used in external ear infections. The infused oil makes an excellent topical antibiotic preparation for festered or infected cuts. You can use it on cuts, scrapes, bruises, and burns to prevent those conditions from becoming infected. The oil may also be used to allay pain in swollen or painful joints by allowing it to be rubbed into and absorbed through the skin. An infusion made of the flowers can be used as a mild sedative. Leaves: have an expectorant property, also a mucilagenic effect. You may use Mullein in either by itself or you can use in combinations for lower respiratory problems such as bronchitis, pneumonia, whooping cough, etc. It can be used alone or mixed with Lobelia to purify and purge the lymphatic system when there is long term glandular swelling.

Dosage >
    Capsules: 4-8 "0" capsules 3x daily.
    Infusion: 1 cup of tea 4x daily.
    Oil: As needed.

Myrrh >

Latin description: Commithora molmol.

Parts to use: Gum / resin.

Chemical constituents: Volatile oil, heerabolene, limonene, eugenol, cinamalhyde, cuminaldehyde, resins, dipentene.

Applications and uses: Myrrh is a beneficial herb to include in mouthwashes and gargles. It is an antiseptic, antifungal and it stimulates your immune, and circulatory systems. Because of its antiseptic, antifungal, and astringent properties it is a beneficial topical cleanser for cleaning out sores and abscesses. Myrrh is also good for preventing infections in scrapes and burns. Myrrh is used for washing wounds and for external or topical skin diseases. I have found it good when mixed with Goldenseal and salt and snuffing it up the nostrils to clear out sinus infections. Myrrh may be used internally for candida albicans and externally for athletes foot. It is excellent for cleansing the mouth of oral ulcers, trench mouth, thrush, pyorrhea, etc. It can also be used internally for purifying mucous in the intestines. Internally myrrh is a mild expectorant.
CAUTION: Avoid long term use.

Dosage >
Capsules: 1-5 "0" capsules 3x daily.

Infusion: Drink 1/2 cup 3x daily.

Nettle > Also known as: Stinging nettles, roman nettles.

Latin description: Urtica dioica.

Parts to use: Aerial.

Chemical constituents: Formic acid, histamine, acetylcholine, chlorine, chlorophyll iodine, tannins, a very
broad spectrum of trace minerals, glucoquinones, 5-
hydroxytryptamine, serotonin.

Applications and uses: Stinging nettles is used as a blood
tonic and cleanser. They are excellent in dealing with
rheumatism and gout as they increases the excretion of
the uric acid in the urine. Because of the wide range
and generous proportions of trace minerals they would
be excellent to include in the diet where ever remineral-
ization would be necessary. Of course nettles would
be indicated for degenerative or osteo arthritis. The
infusion is excellent in cleansing the urinary system in
cases of urinary infections or cystitis. Because of the
acetylcholine and serotonin it would be indicated to use
for insomnia, chronic depression, and a post recupera-
tive for head or brain injuries. Nettles may be beneficial
to use for schizophrenia. Nettles can be used to
counteract anemia due to the blending ratio of the
vitamin C and iron they contain. An infusion can be
used externally for rinses for the scalp and hair to
increase the vitality and life of both. It is indicated in
cases of scalp conditions such as dandruff. It is also a
good wash for eczema. Nettles may also be used for a
poultice, plaster or compress directly on painful joints
due to arthritis. Nettles will increase the flow of breast

milk in lactating mothers. They may be used effectively in diabetes to lower blood sugar levels. They can be made into an astringent for bleeding. The infusion may be injected vaginally to stop excess bleeding in menstruation. If used with Mullein, Comfrey, or Lobelia an infusion is good to eradicate excess phlegm from the lungs. Some herbalists recommend either the infusion or the fresh juice to the scalp for baldness.

Dosage >
Capsules: 3-8 "0" capsules 3x daily.
Infusion: 2-3 ounces as needed up to 4x daily.

Oregon Grape > Also known as: Rocky mountain grape, mountain grape, holly leaf, California barberry.

Latin description: Berberis aquifolium or mahoniaa aquifolium.

Parts to use: Rhizome and root.

Chemical constituents: Berberine, berbamine, herbamine, oxyacanthine.

Applications and uses: A highly effective blood and tissue cleanser. Because of its bitter properties it can be used to stimulate the liver and gallbladder function. Oregon grape stimulates the production of bile, consequently it is an excellent digestive tonic. Use would be indicated wherever one would notice skin eruptions and skin impurities, typically with any type of skin disorder. If dealing with a life threatening disease such as cancer or other conditions it would be the best purifier for the blood, tissues, and body to allow the immune system to function properly. Also indicated use for rheumatism if you don't have other herbs as it is not the very first choice. It can also be used in conditions of hypothyroidism to stimulate the thyroid. As we see Goldenseal become extinct, Oregon grape may become a substitute. Use 3 parts Oregon grape, and 1 part Echinacea Angustifolia instead of Goldenseal. **CAUTION:** Since it does contain Berberine, which is a uterine stimulator, it should be avoided during pregnancy unless taken under the advice of a qualified practitioner. It could cause a spontaneous abortion.

Dosage>
    Capsules: 4 "0" capsules 3x daily.
    Decoction: 3 ounces 3x daily.

Parsley >

Latin description: Petroselinum crispum

Parts to use: Leaves, roots, and seeds.

Chemical constituents: Apiin, apiol, bergaptein, myristicin, pinene, flavonoids, glycoside, camphor, petrocelinic acid, furanocumarin, iodine, Vitamin C, A, iron, manganese, calcium, and phosphorus, chlorophyll.

Applications and uses: Parsley is a powerful urinary cleanser. Sometimes when combined with other herbs such as yarrow it is excellent in treating urinary infections. It is good for the entire urinary tract. Parsley aids in uric acid elimination and would be indicated in conditions of rheumatoid arthritis, gout, etc. It is good for thyroid malfunction. It helps to eliminate intestinal gas. It is a digestive tonic. It sweetens the breath and is a recommended remedy for anemia. The root is good specifically in dealing with liver disorders especially jaundice. The seeds are recommended for amenorrhea or dysmenorrhea and regulating menstrual cycles. Parsley has a tremendous amount of chlorophyll. Cancerous cells find great difficulty in multiplying in the presence of parsley. It can be eaten freely however, it does block vitamin B-12 absorption. It is a beneficial uterine muscle toner and could be used postpartum to get back in shape. **CAUTION:** It should not be used in therapeutic doses during pregnancy.

Dosage >
Capsules: 4 "0" capsules 4x daily.
Infusion: 4-6 ounces up to 4x daily.

Pau D'Arco > Also known as: Taheebo.

Latin description: Tabebuia heptaphylla.

Parts to use: Inner bark.

Chemical constituents: Lapachol.

Applications and uses: Pau D'Arco has antibacterial, antifungal, and antiviral properties. It is beneficial in candida albicans. Antifungal tinctures are good for infections in nail beds. It is useful in thrush as a decoction. It is very useful as a douche in vaginal yeast infections. It is widely used in South America as a cancer remedy due to its antiviral and anticancer action. **CAUTION:** Avoid use where weakened kidneys are involved. Avoid long term use.

Dosage >
Capsules: 4-6 "0" capsules 2x daily.
Decoction: Drink 2 cups daily.

Peppermint > Also known as: Mint.

Latin description: Mentha piperita.

Parts to use: Aerial and tender stems.

Chemical constituents: Menthol, menthone, menthylacetate, menthofuran, tanic acid, terpenes, limonene, pulegone, cineole, bisabolene, isomenthol, neomenthol, phytol, tocopherol, carotenoid, betane, choline.

Applications and uses: Peppermint contains a mild anti-spasmodic therefore it is good for stomach cramps or colic, and is good for dispelling intestinal gas. It is a digestive tonic, it increases the appetite, and increases the flow of bile. Peppermint has been shown to be effective in healing ulcers. The oil is antibacterial and can be used externally. It is also antiparasitic and can be used internally with caution. The oil can be used externally also in relieving pain and can be included in massage oils and liniments. Peppermint oil will greatly increase the flow of blood or circulation in the skin where it is applied. The oil can be used to bring circulation to the extremities as in diabetic condition. **CAUTION:** With peppermints possible interference with iron absorption may occur. Oils should not be used on infants. It is not advised to use the oil in steam inhalations.

Dosage >
Capsules: 3 "0" capsules 4x daily.

Infusion: 1 cup 3-4x daily.

Peach >

Latin description: Amygdalus persica.

Parts to use: Leaves and inner bark. The leaf is the most common.

Chemical constituents: Not available.

Applications and uses: Peach leaves taken as an infusion or tincture combat nausea better than any other plant. Large doses may cause diarrhea. It must be used with care as it is also a sedative. It can also be used singularly for a sedative. It also has a sedative effect on intestinal parasites so that they are anesthetized and are passed out of the body.

Dosage>
Capsules: 1-2 caps 3-4x daily.
Infusion: 1/4-1/2 cup 3-4x daily.

Plantain > Also known as: Snake weed, ribwart. There are two types of Plantain.

Latin Description: Plantago major and plantago psyllium.

Parts to use: Plantago Major- leaves. Plantago Psyllium- seeds.

Chemical constituents: Plantago major- leaves- mucilage, tannins, silica. plantago psyllium- higher mucilage, glycosides, monoterpenes, aucubine, enzymes, proteins, fatty acids.

Applications and uses: The leaves can be crushed and applied externally for the pain of stings and insect bites. Internally we use them as a diuretic. Because of the high silica content they are beneficial for poor quality hair or finger and toe nails. Internally for weakened lungs, to help strengthen them. It also has some antibiotic affect. We like to mix it with a raw potato in a juicer and use it in place of antibiotics. Plantain leaf has a tremendous benefit in relieving sinus congestion. Its use would be indicated in sinus infections and sinus headaches. The seeds or Plantago Psyllium-will add bulk to the stools and because of their semi abrasive action they are excellent in bowel cleanses of all types. Typical application involves grinding the seeds. **CAUTION:** If using the psyllium seeds as either a laxative or a bulking agent for the stool it is very important that you not take them in a concentrated form but mix them in juice or water and drink copious amounts of fluid with it. In some cases, predominantly in geriatrics, there have been some reported problems with these seeds clumping and causing obstructions in the bowel.

Dosage >
Leaf -Capsules: 4-6 "0" capsules 4x daily.
Leaf - Infusion 1/2 cup 3x daily.
Leaf - Juice 1 teaspoon to 1 tablespoon 4x daily.
Seed Powder: 1 rounded teaspoon mixed in 8 oz.
    of juice or water. Mix well before drinking.

Pleurisy Root > Also known as: Canada root, tuber root.

Latin description: Asclepias tuberosa.

Parts to use: Root.

Chemical constituents: Glycosides, volatile oil, resin.

Applications and uses: It's name implies that it is indicated for use in pleurisy. It is an expectorant and a diaphoretic. Pleurisy root may also be used for pneumonia. It is sometimes used in a decoction for gastric irritability. It can be used orally and also as a high enema since it is cleansing and also soothing to the irritation. Decoctions are also useful in asthma. **CAUTION:** High doses can be emetic in nature.

Dosage >
Capsules: 4 "0" capsules 3x daily.
Decoction: 1 cup 3x daily.

Poke Root > Also known as : Pigeon berry, poke.

Latin description: Phytolacca americana.

Parts to use: Root.

Chemical constituents: Triterpenoid saponins, phytolaccine, phytolaccic acid, tannins, resins.

Applications and uses: Poke is cleansing to the lymphatic system. It is also a powerful bowel cleanser and tissue cleanser. Poultices may be used for a wide variety of infections and inflammatory processes. Some of the substances that it contains have been highly beneficial in dealing with AIDS and other retro viruses. Typically, those who treat these kinds of things are using the fresh leaves, the more tender part of the leaves in the earlier part of the year. The chemical constituents of the poke plant are said to be 1,000 times more beneficial against AIDS than AZT. It is also used by many natural practitioners in treating cancer. It is indicated in use for swollen breasts from mastitis used as a poultice and also is beneficial in treating fibroids.

CAUTION: Do not eat the berries. In using the fresh leaves you MUST know what you are doing. If you get the wrong maturity of leaf you can have a toxic or even a fatal effect.

Dosage >
   Capsules: up to 2 "0" capsules 3x daily.
   Decoction: 1/2 cup 3x daily. Use with caution. There is no dosage given for the fresh plant as you must know what you are doing with this part personally.

Red Clover >

Latin description: Trifolium pratense.

Part to use: Dried flowers.

Chemical constituents: Coumarins, phenolic glycosides, flavonoids, salicylates, inositol, cyanogenic glycosides.

Applications and uses: Red clover is of great benefit in stimulating and supporting the immune system. It is an excellent blood purifier, especially when mixed with grape juice. It has a very mild sedative effect, and is a mild expectorant. It is good for bronchial inflammation. Clover has demonstrable anticancer properties.

Dosage >
   Capsules: 4-6 "0" capsules 4x daily.
   Infusion: Drink freely.

Red Raspberry >

Latin description: Rubus idaeus.

Parts to use: Leaves.

Chemical constituents: Citric acid, silicon, fragarine, tannins.

Applications and uses: Raspberry leaf is a refrigerant and is used to cool excessive fevers. It may diminish menstrual bleeding. It tones the uterus during pregnancy. Raspberry is typically not recommended for pregnancy unless taken during the last trimester. It also is beneficial in stimulating lactation. The leaf internally acts as an astringent and does help to allay the symptoms of diarrhea. The infusion has been used at times as a mouth wash or an oral wash or gargle to relieve and heal sores in the mouth and oral tissues. It should not be taken in large quantities such as more than one quart of tea daily for long periods such as more than two weeks. If taken in large quantities for extended periods of time it blocks iron absorption which could cause anemia.

Dosage>
Capsules: 3 caps 3-4x daily.
Infusion: 1 cup 3x daily.

Shepherds Purse > Also known as: Witch pouch, pick pocket.

Latin Description: Capsella bursa-pastoris.

Parts to use: Ariel.

Chemical Constituents: Acetyl choline, tyramine.

Applications and uses: Because it is an astringent it is used
in case of chronic or profuse diarrhea. Shepherds
purse is a very effective diuretic. It is cleansing to the
urinary tract. It can be made into a compress or poultice and used for hemorrhoids and external bleeding
ulcers. The infusion may be snuffed to halt nose bleeds.

Dosage >
Capsules: 4 caps 2x daily.
Infusion: 1 cup 2x daily.

Sarsaparilla >

Latin description: Smilax ornata or smilax officinalis.

Parts to use: Root.

Chemical constituents: Glycosides, steroids, steroidal
saponins, essential oil, parillin resin, sarsaponin,
sitosterol, stigmasterin.

Applications and uses: Sarsaparilla cleanses and purifies
the blood. It is indicated for cleansing the blood in
situations of skin diseases and will clear up skin disorders such as acne, psoriasis, and possibly eczema.
Because of the steroidal components it can reduce the
pain of arthritis. It is also a diaphoretic and makes it
excellent in causing sweats. A carminative for reducing
intestinal gas. Sarsaparilla is used in regulating hormone
balance.

Dosage >
Capsules: 4 "0" capsules 3x daily.

Decoction: 1/2 cup 3x daily.

Scullcap >

Latin description: Scutellaria literifolia.

Parts to use: Aerial.

Chemical constituents: Tannins, volatile oil, flavonoid glycosides.

Applications and uses: It is a nervine and has a tonic effect on the nervous system. Scullcap can help in controlling epilepsy. Scullcap is indicated with head aches of any type. It may also be used in insomnia, nervousness and depression. This herb can improve circulation, so could help with migraine headaches.
CAUTION: Do not take large doses and avoid long term use. Do not use for people who have a history of erratic heart rate.

Dosage >
Capsules: 2 "0" capsules 3x daily.
Infusion: 1/2 - 1 cup 2-3x daily.

Skunk Cabbage > Also known as: Meadow cabbage, pole cat weed.

Latin description: Symplocarpus foetidus.

Parts to use: Root.

Chemical constituents: Silica, iron, volatile oil, resin.

Applications and uses: In addition to it's unpleasant odor it

has some sedative and antispasmodic properties. It is
useful in herbal combinations for asthma and seizure
disorders and has been traditionally used effectively
against whooping cough. There is a possibility for it to
be used also for either bronchitis or pleurisy.

Dosage >
    Capsules: 2 "0" capsules every 4 hours.
    Decoction: Do not use the fresh root, it should be
      dried. 1/4 cup as needed.

Slippery Elm > Also known as: Red elm, moose elm, Indian
elm, sweet elm.

Latin description: Ulmus fulva

Parts to use: Inner bark.

Chemical constituents: Mucilage, phosphorus, polysaccharides, tannins, starch.

Applications and uses: Slippery Elm is quite soothing in
cases of internal inflammation, especially in the gastrointestinal tract. It is indicated in diarrhea and is very
useful for ulcers and ulcerative colitis as it not only
coats but heals. Slippery elm can also be used as a
substitute for eggs in the culinary field for its binding
ability. Many herbalists use the powdered bark as a
binder in making pills and herbal preparations. It is an
excellent material to use in poultices as it is very soothing but it is drawing also.

Dosage >
    Capsules: 4-8 "0" capsules 3-4x daily.
    Decoction: 1 cup 3-4x daily.

Sorrell Grass > Also known as: Sour grass, incorrectly called sheep sorrell.

Latin description: Oxalis acetosella.

Parts to use: Leaves.

Chemical constituents: Potassium, oxalate, oxalic acid, mucilage.

Applications and uses: In culinary usage it may be used to replace vinegar. Its primary use and most important is as an escharotic. Natural practitioners use the leaves in removing skin cancers and small external tumors. It may be used internally as an anticancer agent, with caution, possibly using licorice as a buffer. Follow up with parsley to expel any of the acids after internal use.

Dosage >
Capsules: 4 caps 2x daily.
Infusion: 1 cup 2x daily, not used internally very often.

St. John's Wort >

Latin description: Hypericum perforatum.

Parts to use: Aerial.

Chemical constituents: Hypericin, flavonoids, tannin, volatile oil, pigment, resin.

Applications and uses: Recent research has revealed that hypericin is very effective in controlling retro-viruses such as AIDS and chronic fatigue. It has long been established as an effective remedy for neuralgia. Many natural practitioners prescribe St. John's wort for the condition of sciatica. The infused oil is excellent for a topical application for injuries and wounds due to its antibacterial action, also for its sedative properties. It is not only soothing but is quite healing and protects against infection. St. John's wort is an effective anti-depressant and is used to level mood swings and calm nervousness. It has been used by some to allay the pain with menstrual cramps. It is a mild diuretic.

Dosage >
Capsules: 3-4 "0" capsules 3-4x daily.
Infusion: 1-2 ounces at a time throughout the day. For a therapeutic dose you may take up to 2-3 cups but NOT for long term, for a few days only! unless you are dealing with a condition such as AIDS where it would take advanced dosages for an extended length of time and should only be done under the supervision of an experienced practitioner.

Valerian > Also known as: All-heal, setwall.

Latin description: Valeriana officinalis.

Parts to use: Root.

Chemical constituents: acidic acid, butyric acid, isovalerianic acid, limonene, camphene, chatinine, choline, fvalerine, valeric acid, alkaloids, valtrate, didovaltrate, valerosidatum, volatile oils, sesquiter pene, pinene, formic acid, tannins, resins.

Applications and uses: Valerian root is a very useful nervine. It can be used for headaches, muscle pain, nervous tension, insomnia, convulsions, muscle cramps, muscle spasms. Some practitioners find it good in controlling palpitations of the heart. It has long been used to lower blood pressure due to hypertension and can improve circulation. It is effective in relieving menstrual cramps and can also help to relieve spastic bowel syndrome. **CAUTION:** Avoid large doses and long term usage. It is possible to become dependant upon it.

Dosage >
Capsules: 2 "0" capsules 3x daily.
Decoction: Take no more than 3 ounces 3x daily.
This is not a starting dosage but should be started at a lower dosage and work up to this.

Vervain > Also known as: Blue vervain.

Latin description: Verbena officinalis.

Parts to use: Aerial.

Chemical constituents: Glycosides, tannins, verbenalian, verbenin, alkaloid, volatile oils.

Applications and uses: It is effective in treating migraines and other headaches of nervous types. Vervain be cause of its bitter properties has a purging or purifying effect on both the liver or gallbladder. The glycosides will help to bring on delayed menses. It does have a mild diaphoretic. It can help to ease labor by encouraging contractions. Vervain has a mild antihistamine effect and is good for colds and sinus disorders. **CAUTION:** Avoid use during pregnancy as it has a uterine stimulator.

Dosage >
    Capsules: 3-4 "0" capsules 3x daily.
    Infusion: up to 1 cup 3x daily.

Violet > Also known as: Blue violet, sweet violet.

Latin description: Viola odorata.

Parts to use: Leaves, flowers, roots.

Chemical constituents: Methyl salicylates, alkaloids,
    volatile oil, flavonoids, saponins.

Applications and uses: The leaves have long been used as a
    cancer treatment for natural practitioners. They have
    some positive effects for fighting cancerous tumors.
    The leaves are also somewhat of a refrigerant and can
    be used in cooling fevers and profuse sweating. The
    root is an emetic in large doses. The flowers have a
    slight sedative. You can make a tea of violet flowers for
    either nervous tension or insomnia.

Dosage >
    Capsules: Leaf only- 3 "0" capsules 3x daily.
    Decoction: Root - Typically 1-2 cups will cause
        vomiting and is used as an emetic
    Infusion: Leaves- 1/2 cup 2-3x daily. It is best to start
        low and work up to your level as sometimes the tea
        from leaves can cause nausea in higher doses.
        Flowers - up to 1 cup as needed as a sedative.

White Birch > Also known as: Paper birch.

Latin description: Betula alba.

Parts to use: Leaves, inner bark and light twigs.

Chemical constituents: Volatile oils, saponins, flavonoids, hyperosid, resins, tannins, sesquiterpenes, betuloventic acid.

Applications and uses: Infusions of the twigs and bark are good for fevers and act as refrigerant. It can be used as a skin wash in skin disorders. Infusions of the leaves are used to promote the growth of hair in early baldness. It is cleansing for dandruff. It is very cleansing in cases of urinary tract infection and inflammation. The greatest known use is in dissolving kidney stones and urinary gravel. To dissolve kidney stones, use an infusional decoction of the leaves and twigs. Better results are obtained by the addition of gravel root, hydrangea, and parsley leaf.

Dosage >
Capsules: 3 "0" capsules 3x daily.
Decoction: Bark & twigs - 1 cup as needed.
Infusion: Leaves - 3 cups daily.

White Oak >

Latin description: Quercus alba.

Parts to use: Inner bark.

Chemical constituents: Tannins, sodium sulphur, calcium, abundance of trace minerals, also Vit B-12! gallic acid, ellagitannin.

Applications and uses: A decoction of the bark is an
    excellent astringent. It also is good in purging intestinal
    parasites. The tannins anesthetize them and they are
    passed out. It is a tremendous healing agent as a com-
    press or wash for wounds. White oak decoction used
    as a compress will lessen the pain from most open
    wounds. It works even better if combined with com-
    frey leaf. It helps to cleanse the puss out of wounds
    and prevents infection due to its astringent action.
    Gargling is great for sore throats. In cases of extreme
    constipation you may use a large glass of the decoction
    orally followed with a high enema of very warm decoc-
    tion. It is very effective to use in bowel cleanses by
    increasing the parastolic action of the colon. It is an
    excellent cleanser and is better in my opinion than
    coffee for that application. The decoction can be used
    in case of diarrhea to stop chronic diarrhea. It is a
    good application for irritable bowel syndrome as it
    helps to cleanse the mucous out of the colon. Because
    of the astringent effect it will help to stop internal bleed-
    ing. It is good for bleeding ulcers. It works well as a
    compress for varicose veins. White oak bark decoc-
    tion is also good in purging the liver and helps to expel
    gall stones. Use it as a wash for pyorrhea and other
    oral inflammations.

Dosage >
    Capsules: up to 8 "0" capsules as needed.
    Decoction: up to 8 ounces at one time if needed,
        although that would only be for an extreme case of
        constipation. 1-2 ounces at a time may be used for
        bleeding ulcers.

White Willow > Also known as: Willow.

Latin description: Salix alba.

Parts to use: Bark.

Chemical constituents: Tannins, salicylic glycosides.

Applications and uses: Due to the salicylic glycosides, white willow can be used effectively as an antiinflammatory/analgesic. Because it is balanced by tannins it does not cause stomach upset or gastric irritation like an aspirin would where the salicylic compounds have been isolated. Typical usages would be where anyone would want to use aspirin. It also works well as a gargle for sore throats. Drinking the decoction also will help to take the inflammation out of urinary tract infections.

Dosage >
Capsules: 4-5 "0" capsules as needed.
Decoction: 1 cup as needed.

Wild Yam > Also known as: Wild Mexican yam.

Latin description: Dioscorea villosa.

Parts to use: Root and rhizome.

Chemical constituents: Steroidal saponins, tannins, phytosterols, dioscorea, starch.

Applications and uses: Wild yam has gained wide acceptance as a hormone balancer due to its dioscorea content. Dioscorea is the precursor for the body to make DHEA. It is indicated in use for irregular menstruation. It eases the symptoms of PMS and menopause. It has some antispasmodic properties and is beneficial in dealing with restless leg syndrome, neuralgias, charley horses, etc. It also helps to increase circulation. The antiinflammatory side of it makes it desirable in dealing with arthritis. It is a mild digestive tonic. It has recently been proven to be beneficial in helping to scavenge arterial plaque in cases of arteriosclerosis. It helps to prevent miscarriage. Wild yam can help over come infertility. NOTE: Yams (dioscorea) and sweet potatoes (ipomoea batatas) are NOT in the same botanical family. The tubers sold in grocery stores as yams are not yams at all, they are sweet potatoes! Wild yam is not related at all to the sweet potato family.

Dosage >
Capsules: 4 caps 3x daily.
Decoction: 1 cup 3x daily.

Witch Hazel > Also known as: Spotted alder, snapping hazelnut, winterbloom.

Latin description: Hamamelis virginiana.

Parts to use: Bark and sometimes leaves.

Chemical constituents: Gallotanins, proanthocyanidins, saponins, choline, resins, flavonoids, volatile oil.

Applications and uses: Astringent, therefore it is helpful in stopping excessive bleeding. It makes a good wash for oral sores or infections. Also a decoction is excellent in cleansing infected eyes especially with conjunctivitis. Because of its chemical constituents of proanthocyanidins there is potential as a free radical scavenger and possibly would be indicated for use with some forms of arthritis as an anti-inflammatory and may be used internally or externally.

Dosage >
Capsules: Bark- 3-4 "0" capsules 2-3x daily.
Decoction: Bark- 1-2 cups daily.
Infusion: Leaves- 1/2 cup 3x daily.

Yarrow > Also known as: Millefoil, nosebleed, thousandleaf.

Latin description: Achillea millefolium.

Parts to use: Aerial, especially the flowering heads.

Chemical constituents: Isovalerianic acid, salicylic acid, asparagin, achilleine, cyanidin, camphor, azulene, borneol, terpineol, cineole, sterols, flavonoids, lactones, isoartemesia ketone, sucrose, mannitol.

Applications and uses: Yarrow is an excellent flu remedy. A hot infusion will produce a nice therapeutic sweat and will help to expel the toxic chemicals out through the sweat or perspiration. It will eventually in long term use cool the body. The infusion is helpful to treat rheumatism and rheumatoid arthritis. It has anti-inflammatory salicylic acid and cyanidin. Compresses of the infusion may be applied to stop bleeding and to heal wounds. Yarrow is very beneficial and useful to regulate heart beat and also to slow tachycardia. It can be used with equal parts of catnip to quell influenza if done in early stages. It does help to some extent to dilate peripheral arteries and vessels and may in short term possibly help to lower blood pressure. In a compress externally it has terrific antiseptic properties. The infusion is an excellent vaginal douche or enema to purify and stop hemorrhaging. It will also help to alleviate pain in the bowel when used as an enema. **CAUTION:** Possible photo sensitivity from internal use but very unlikely.

Dosage >
    Capsules: 6-8 "0" capsules 3x daily.
    Infusion: 1 cup 3x daily.

Yellow Dock > Also known as: Dock.

Latin description: Rumex crispus.

Parts to use: Root.

Chemical constituents: Glycosides, tannins, anthraquinone glycoside, iron.

Applications and uses: Use as an astringent, laxative, liver tonic, blood purifier, and digestive tonic.

Dosage >
    Capsules: 4 caps 3-4x daily.
    Decoction: 1 cup 3x daily.

Glossary of Terms
Used in the Medical Missionary Training Classes

Absorption-Nutritionally, the process by which nutrients are absorbed through the intestinal tract into the bloodstream to be used by the body. If nutrients are not properly absorbed, nutritional deficiencies can result.

Acute illness-An illness that comes on quickly and may cause relatively severe symptoms, but is of limited duration.

Adaptation/adaptogen-These are immune system enhancers which help the body adjust and regulate to restore natural immune resistance.

Aerial -The part of the plant which grows above the ground.

Alterative-These are considered useful in altering the body chemistry. They are blood purifiers which correct impurities in the blood and stimulate gradual changes in metabolism and tissue function in acute and chronic conditions.

Analgesic-These herbs are used to relieve pain.

Anemia-A deficiency in the blood's ability to carry oxygen to the body tissues.

Aneurysm-Localized abnormal dilatation of the blood vessel, usually an artery. Due to congenital defect or weakness of the wall of the vessel.

Angina-Angina pectoris. A syndrome of chest pain with sensations of suffocation, typically brought on by exertion and relieved by rest.

Antibiotic-Herbs that work as natural antibiotics help the body's immune system to destroy both viral and bacterial infections.

Antibody-A protein molecule made by the immune system that is designed to intercept and neutralize a specific invading organism or other foreign substance.

Antidote-Agent which counteracts or destroys the effects of poison or other medicines.

Antigen-A substance that can elicit the formation of an antibody when introduced into the body.

Antihistamine-A substance that interferes with the action of histamines by binding to histamine receptors in various body tissues.

Antioxidant-A substance that blocks or inhibits destructive oxidation reactions. Examples include vitamins C and E, the minerals Selenium and Germanium, the enzymes Catalase and super-oxide dismutase (SOD), coenzyme Q10, and some amino acids.

Antiseptic-Substances that prevent the growth of bacteria.

Antispasmodic-These herbs are used to prevent or counteract spasms.

Aromatic-Agents which emit a gragrant smell and produce a pungent taste. Used chiefly to make other medicines more palatable.

Arteriosclerosis-A circulatory disorder characterized by a thickening and stiffening of the walls of large and medium sized arteries, which impedes circulation.

Auto-immune disorder-Any condition in which the immune system reacts inappropriately to the body's own tissues and attacks them, causing damage and/or interfering with normal functioning. Examples include Bright's disease, diabetes, multiple sclerosis, rheumatoid arthritis, systemic lupus erythematosus.

Astringent-An agent that diminishes internal or external secretions or causes soft tissues to pucker.

Balsamic-A healing or soothing agent.

Benign-Literally, "harmless." Used to refer to cells, especially cells growing in inappropriate locations, that are not malignant (cancerous).

Biopsy-Excision of tissue from a living being for diagnosis.

Bitter tonic-Bitter tasting properties which stimulate the flow of

saliva and gastric juice. Used to increase the appetite
and aid the process of digestion.

Cardiac-Pertaining to the heart.

Cardiac arrhythmia-An abnormal heart rate of rhythm.

Carminatives-Substances used to expel gas from the stomach,
intestines or bowels.

Chemotherapy-Treatment of disease by the use of chemicals
(such as drugs), especially the use of chemical treat-
ments to combat cancer.

Chlorophyll-The pigment responsible for the green color of
plant tissues. It can be taken in supplement form as a
source of magnesium and trace elements.

Chronic illness-A disorder that persists or recurs over an
extended period, often for life. Chronic illness can be
as relatively benign as hay fever or as serious as
multiple sclerosis.

Coagulate-To solidify or to change from a fluid state to a semi-
solid mass, as in blood.

Co-carcinogen-An agent that acts with another to cause
cancer.

Coenzyme-A molecule that works with an enzyme to enable
the enzyme to perform its function in the body. Coen-
zymes are necessary in the utilization of vitamins and
minerals.

Cold-pressed-A term used to describe food oils that are
extracted without the use of heat in order to preserve
nutrients and flavor.

Congenital-Present from birth, but not necessarily inherited.

Contusion-A bruise, an injury in which the skin is not broken.

Decoction-Decoctions are certain preparations made by boiling herbal substances in a covered container in the
amount of one teaspoon per cup of water for a con-
siderable period of time. Hard materials such as roots,
barks, and seeds, are usually prepared in this way as
they require longer subjection to heat (approximately 30

mins.) in order to extract their active principles, then strained and used.

Dementia-A permanent acquired impairment of intellectual function that results in a marked decline in memory, language ability, personality, visuospatial skills, and/or cognition (orientation, perception, reasoning, abstract thinking, and calculation). Dementia can be either static or permanent, and can result from many different causes.

Demulcent-Soothing, bland. Used to relieve internal inflammations. Provides a protective coating and allays irritation of the membranes.

Detoxification-The process of reducing the build-up of various poisonous substances in the body.

Diaphoretic-Substances used to increase perspiration and temperature.

Diuretic-An agent that increases the flow of urine.

Diverticulitis-The inflammation in the intestinal tract especially in the colon, causing stagnation of feces in little distended sacs (diverticula) of the colon and pain.

Edema-Retention of fluid in the tissues that results in swelling.

Electrolyte-Soluble salts dissolved in the body's fluids. Electrolytes are the form in which most minerals circulate in the body. They are so named because they are capable of conducting electrical impulses.

Embolus-A loose particle of tissue, a blood clot, or a tiny air bubble that travels through the blood stream and, if it lodges in a narrowed portion of a blood vessel, can block blood flow.

Emetic-A remedy that induces vomiting.

Emollient-Herbs used externally to help soften, soothe, and protect the skin.

Emulsion-A combination of two liquids that do not mix with each other, such as oil and water; substance is broken into tiny dorplets and is suspended with the other.

Emulsification is the first step in the digestion of fats.

Endemic-Native to or prevalent in a particular geographic region. Often used to describe disease.

Endorphin-One of a number of natural hormonelike substances found primarily in the brain. One function of endorphins is to suppress the sensation of pain, which they do by binding to appropriate receptors in the brain.

Enzymes-Chemical substances, produced by living cells, which speed up the rates of chemical change in our bodies.

Erythema-Reddening, especially of the skin.

Essential Oils-A volatile (easily vaporized) and scented plant oil found in many herbal medications.

Expectorant-Easing the coughing up of mucus.

Extracts-Extracts are made in a variety of ways, depending on the best method by which the plant's properties may be obtained, such as high pressure, evaporation by heat, and the like. Extracts are generally supplied by the various herb companies.

Flatulence-Excessive amounts of gas in the stomach or other parts of the digestive tract.

Flavonoid-Any of a large group of crystalline compounds found in plants.

Fomentations-Local applications of cloths wrung out in hot water, with or without the addition of medicinal agents.

Free radical-An atom or group of atoms that is highly chemically reactive because it has at least one unpaired electron. Because they join so readily with other compounds, free radicals can attack cells and can cause a lot of damage in the body. Free radicals form in heated fats and oils, and as a result of exposure to atmospheric radiation and environmental pollutants, among other things.

Gastritis-Inflammation of the stomach lining.

Gastrointestinal-Pertaining to the stomach, small and large intestines, colon, rectum, liver, pancreas, and gallbladder.

Gingivitis-Inflammation of the gums surrounding the teeth.

Gland-An organ or tissue that secretes a substance(s) for use elsewhere in the body rather than for its own functioning.

Globulin-A type of protein found in the blood. Certain globulins contain disease fighting antibodies.

Glucose-A simple sugar that is the principal source of energy for the body's cells.

Heavy metal-A metallic element whose specific gravity (a measurement of mass as compared with the mass of water or hydrogen) is greater than 5.0. Some heavy metals, such as arsenic, cadmium, lead, and mercury, are extremely toxic.

Hemoglobin-The iron-containing red pigment in the blood that is responsible for the transport of oxygen.

Hemorrhage-Profuse or abnormal bleeding.

Hemostatic-Drugs employed to control bleeding.

Hernia-A condition in which part of an internal organ protrudes, inappropriately, through an opening in the tissues that are supposed to contain it.

Hypertension-High blood pressure. Generally, hypertension is defined as a regular resting pressure over 140/90.

Hypotension-Low blood pressure.

Inflammation-A reaction to illness or injury characterized by swelling, warmth, and redness.

Infusion-Infusions are frequently called teas, and are generally prepared in the amount of one teaspoon herb per cup of water. Usually, the softer substance of the herb such as the blossoms and leaves are prepared as infusions. Boiling water is poured over the herb, the container covered, and the solution allowed to steep for 15 minutes, then strained and used.

Insomnia-The inability to sleep.

Insulin-A hormone produced by the pancreas that regulates the metabolism of glucose (sugar) in the body.

Lactation-The period of suckling in mammals. The function of secreting milk.

Lithotriptic-Herbs which help dissolve and eliminate stones and gravel from the body.

Menorrhea-Normal menstruation.

Malignant-Literally, "evil." Used to refer to cells or groups of cells that are cancerous and likely to spread.

Mitochondria-Tiny structures inside each body cell that produce almost all the energy a cell needs to live and function.

MRI-Magnetic resonance imaging. A technique used in diagnosis that combines the use of radio waves and a strong magnetic field to produce detailed images of the internal structures of the body.

Mucilaginous-A sticky substance found in plants, used to sooth inflammation.

Nervine-An agent which acts on the nervous system to temporarily relax nervous tension or excitement.

Occlude-To close up, obstruct, or join together, as bringing the biting surfaces of opposing teeth together.

Pleurisy-Inflammation of the pleura (portion of the lung).

Poultice-Poultices are made of herbs or charcoal and placed between a gauze-like material with the ends enclosed tightly. This technique is used to draw poisons from the area.

Precursor-Raw materials the body needs to build a substance it naturally requires. With herbal medicines the results may be similar as taking steroids but without the harmful side effects.

Prognosis-A forecast as to the likely course and/or outcome of a disorder or condition.

Purgative-Causes copious evacuations from the bowels. Purgatives are more drastic than laxatives or aperients, and are generally combined with other agents to control or modify their action.

Refrigerant-Relieves thirst and produces a sensation of coolness.

Retrovirus-A type of virus that has RNA as its core nucleic acid and contains an enzyme called reverse transcriptase that permits the virus to copy its RNA into the DNA of infected cells, in effect taking over the cells' genetic machinery. Human immunodeficiency virus (HIV), the virus that causes AIDS, is a retrovirus. Retroviruses are also known to cause certain types of cancer in animals, and are suspected of causing forms of leukemia and lymphoma in humans.

Rhizome-A rootlike stem growing horizontal along or below the ground and sending out roots and shoots.

Sedative-Calms the nerves.

Steroid-One of a group of fat-soluble organic compounds with a characteristic chemical composition. A number of different hormones, drugs, and other substances-including cholesterol-are classified as steroids.

Stimulant-Increases or quickens various functional actions of the system.

Systemic-Pertaining to the entire body.

Tannin-Acid substance found in bark of certain plants and trees or their products, usually from nutgall.

T cell-A type of lymphocyte that is a crucial part of the immune system.

Tincture-Tinctures are spirituous preparations made with pure or diluted alcohol (usually Vodka). Tinctures are employed because some herbs will not yield their properties with water alone, or may be rendered useless by applications of heat. Generally, the herb/herbs are placed in a glass jar with Vodka completely covering them and the lid tightly closed. The herbs are allowed to soak for at least two weeks and the jar is shaken daily. Then the herbs are strained out and the "tincture" is what remains. The alcohol may be removed from the herbal medicine by putting in a swallow or two of boiling water and let sit for 10 minutes.

Tonic-Herbs used to increase tone, energy, vigor and strength by nourishing the body.

Toxin-A poison that impairs the health and functioning of the body.

Trace element-A mineral required by the body in extremely small quantities.

Tremor-Involuntary trembling.

Vascular-Pertaining to the circulatory system.

Vermifuge-Expels or destroys worms.

Vital signs-Basic indicators of an individual's health status, including pulse, respirations, blood pressure, and body temperature.

Useful Abbreviations

b.i.d.-two times per day.

t.i.d.-three times per day.

q.i.d.-four times per day.

p.r.n.-as needed.

Index

A

Abrasions 16, 17, 58, 59
Abscess 34, 59
Acne 23, 41, 70
ADD-Attention Deficit 38, 46
Adrenal
  Function 18
AIDS 67, 74
Allergic Reaction 54
Allergies 57
Alzhiemers 42
Amenorrhea 63
Anemia 60, 62, 69
Angina 47
Antiangiogenic. *See also* Cancer
Antibacterial 17, 19, 26, 27, 31, 42, 44, 63, 64, 74
Antibiotic 32, 34, 41, 44, 58, 66
Antidepressant 36, 74
Antiemetic 29
Antifungal 30, 41, 42, 44, 45, 59, 63
Antihistamine 36, 75
Antiinflammatory 20, 24, 25, 29, 30, 31, 40, 44, 54, 79, 80, 81
Antimicrobial 23
Antiseptic 37, 51, 53, 59, 81
Antispasmodic 20, 21, 24, 30, 49, 55, 64, 72, 79
Antiviral 25, 27, 34, 36, 44, 63
Appetite
  Stimulant 21, 25, 64
Arterial plaque 41, 42, 80
Arteriosclerosis 24
Arthritis 19, 20, 21, 26, 29, 43, 46, 53, 54, 60, 70, 80, 81
  Osteo 23, 40, 60
  Rheumatoid 20, 23, 38, 40, 62, 81

94

Asthma 20, 29, 35, 36, 40, 48, 55, 67, 72
Astringent 39, 59, 61, 69, 70, 78, 80, 82
Athletes foot 41, 59

B

B-12 63, 77
Bad Breath 62
Birthing 22
Bites 34, 66
Bleeding 17, 26, 50, 58, 61, 70, 78, 81
  Excessive 80
Blood 34
  Builder 34
  Coagulant 50
  Purifier 22, 27, 39, 45, 60, 61, 68, 70, 82
  Thinner 41
Blood Pressure 36, 47
  High 22, 24, 26, 32, 36, 41, 45, 47, 48, 57, 75, 81
  Low 47
Blood Sugar
  High 41, 61
  Low 23
Boils 23, 34, 40
Bone
  Growth 30
  Spurs 23
Bowel cleanse 66, 67, 78
Brain
  Function 42
  Injury 46, 60
Bronchial Inflammation 68
Bronchitis 21, 29, 31, 35, 43, 51, 58, 72
Bruises 30, 55, 58
Burns 16, 31, 58, 59

C

Cancer 26, 27, 31, 41, 61, 63, 68, 73, 76
Candida Albicans 41, 59, 63
Cartilage
  Production 30
Cataracts 39

Chemical Toxicity 27, 38, 56, 81
Cholesterol 41, 47
Chronic Fatigue 18, 74
Circulation 24, 42, 48, 59, 64, 71, 75, 80
Colds 25, 36, 48, 75
Colic 25, 64
Colitis 49, 72
Congestion 43, 66
  Nasal 39, 59
Conjunctivitis 29, 39, 80
Constipation 16, 19, 23, 66, 78
Convulsions 75
Cough 29, 37, 48, 56
Cramps
  Menstrual 20, 21, 33, 46, 49, 74, 75
  Muscle 75
  Stomach 21, 25, 49, 64
Crohns 25
Cuts 17, 58
Cystitis 23, 53, 60

D

Dandruff 32, 60, 77
Decongestant 36, 39
Deodorant 32
Depression 45, 49, 60, 71
Dermatitis 28
Diabetes 24, 41, 45, 61, 64
Diarrhea 17, 21, 25, 41, 47, 65, 69, 70, 72, 78
Digestive
  Aid 25, 34, 44, 61, 62, 64, 80, 82
  Irritant 26
Digestive System 18
Diptheria 41
Diuretic 18, 21, 23, 32, 34, 45, 46, 50, 53, 66, 70, 74
Dysmenorrhea 21, 36, 63

E

Ear
  Ache 41
  Infection 41, 58

Eczema 23, 28, 60, 70
Emetic 21, 55, 67, 76
Epilepsy 38, 55, 71
Expectorant 29, 35, 41, 48, 51, 56, 58, 59, 67, 68
Eyes 29, 39, 44, 80, 82
    Weak 39

F

Fevers 32, 50, 55, 69, 77
Fibroids 28, 68
Flu 25, 36, 81
Fluid Retention 25
Food Poison 44
Free Radicals 27, 80

G

Gallbladder 23, 61, 75, 78
Gargle 17, 26, 59, 69, 78, 79
Gas 48, 62, 64, 70
Gastrointestinal tract 16, 52, 56, 67, 72
    ulcers 44
Glaucoma 36
Gout 46, 53, 60, 62

H

Hair 50, 60, 77
Hayfever 29, 36, 39
Headache 29, 71, 75
    Migraine 40, 71, 75
Heart
    Attack 26, 47
    Congestive Failure 45
    Disease 22, 42
    Function 45, 47
    Rapid rate 19, 33, 47, 57, 81
    Regulate 42, 71, 75, 81
    Thrombosis 36
Hemorrhaging. *See also* Bleeding
Hemorrhoids 42, 70
Hepatitis 41, 56

Herpes 36
Herpes Simplex Virus 51
Hormone
   Balance 28, 70, 79
   Hot flashes 39
Hypoglycemia 23

I

Immune System 18, 23, 25, 34, 41, 59, 61, 68
Infections 31, 34, 41, 59, 67, 74, 78
Infertility 80
Inflammation 19, 67
Insomnia 25, 29, 45, 47, 49, 60, 71, 75, 76
Irritable Bowel Syndrome. *See also* Colitis

J

Jaundice 63
Joints 17, 21, 58
   Pain 60

K

Kidney
   Cleanse 43
   Problems 53
   Stones 46, 77
   Weak 63

L

Labor 22, 57, 75
Lactation 21, 39, 61, 69
Laxative 16, 19, 23, 66, 82
Leprosy 45
Lice 37
Liver 31, 63
   Cleanse 19, 23, 34, 39, 44, 57, 75, 78, 83
   Function 27, 45, 61
   Restore 21, 23, 34, 36, 37, 56
Lock jaw 55
Lungs 37
   Congested 29

Inflammation 21
Mucous 61
Lymph
Cleanse 32, 50, 67
Swollen 34

M

Mastitis 68
Memory 42, 46
Meningitis 55
Menopause 28, 39, 49, 57, 79
Menstration
Excessive 28
Menstrual
Bleeding 69
Cramps 21, 33, 46, 49, 74, 75
Flow 28
Regulate 28, 49, 57, 63, 79
Menstruation
Delayed 75
Excessive 45, 50, 61
Metabolic
Function 19
Migraine 40, 46, 71, 75
Miscarriage 33, 80
Mood swings 74
Mouth 17, 26, 39, 44, 51, 69, 78, 79, 80
Mucous 31, 59
Membranes 44
Multiple Sclerosis 38
Muscle
Cramps 75
Pain 75
Relaxant 33
Spasms 21, 54
Sprains 55

N

Nails 44, 50, 63
Nausea 65
Nervine 29, 49, 55, 71, 75

Nervous 49, 71, 74, 75, 76
Neuopathy 24
Neuralgia 54, 74, 80
Nose Bleeds 70
Nursing 20, 39, 60, 69

O

Obesity 19, 80
Oral sores/ulcers 17, 26, 41, 44, 51, 59, 69, 79, 80

P

Pain 20, 40, 49, 58
  Abdominal 47
  Bowel 82
  Joint 17, 60
  Topical 54
  Wounds 78
Parasites 27, 35, 41, 52, 64, 65, 78
Pelvic Inflammation 46
Phlebitis 24
Pink Eye 39
Pleurisy 21, 26, 43, 67, 72
PMS 28, 38, 79
Pneumonia 43, 51, 55, 58, 67
Poultices 31, 34
Pregnancy 33, 69
  Cautions 22, 40, 45, 58, 62, 63, 75
  Difficulties 33
Prostate
  Enlargement 36
  Inflammation 32, 45, 46, 50
Psoriasis 23, 28, 70
Pulmonary
  Infection 35
Pyorrhea 59, 78

R

Reproduction 28
Respiratory
  Congestion 29, 43

Disorders 20, 31, 36, 51, 58, 64
Infection 35, 43
Restless Leg Syndrome 80
Rheumatism 19, 29, 46, 53, 54, 60, 61, 81
Ringworm 44

S

Scabies 36
Schizophrenia 60
Scrapes 16, 17, 58
Sedative 20, 25, 49, 58, 65, 68, 72, 74, 76
Seizures 72
Sinuses 31, 39, 59, 66, 75
Skin
    Cancer 73
    Disorders 23, 37, 38, 44, 50, 59, 61, 70, 77
    Infections 23
Smoking 50, 55
Sore throat 17, 26, 78, 79
Sores 40, 41, 54, 59
Spasms 24, 75
    Muscle 21
Spastic colon. *See also* Colitis
Spleen
    Enlarged 19
Staph 30
Stomach
    Upset 25
Stones
    Gall 78
    Kidney 46, 77
    Urinary 32, 43, 50, 56, 77
Stress 49
Stroke 41
Sunburn 16
Sweats 18, 21, 25, 36, 51, 67, 70, 75, 76, 81
Swelling 19
    Glands 58

T

Thrombosis 24

Thrush 30, 44, 59, 63
Thyroid 19, 62
  Hyperthyroidism 36
  Hypothyroidism 62
Tissue 44
  Cleanse 23, 27, 61, 67
  Growth 30
Tuberculosis 35, 41, 45
Tumors 73, 76
Typhoid 41

U

Ulcers 18, 31, 44, 52, 56, 64, 70, 72, 78
Urinary
  Cleanse 27, 32, 43, 53, 60, 62, 70
  Cystitis 53, 60
  Infection 32, 46, 53, 56, 60, 62, 77, 79
  Problems 23
  Stones 32, 43, 50, 56, 77

V

Vaginal 81
  Infections 44, 53, 63
Varicose veins 31, 42, 78

W

Wash 30, 35, 39, 51, 53, 59, 69, 77, 78, 80,
Whooping cough 20, 30, 36, 58, 72
Wounds 54, 74, 78, 81

Y

Yeast 44, 54, 64

Notes

Notes

Now is the TIME to Know

The Bible is as relevant as ever to your life and family. Let us prove it! Our Bible Study Guides will help you understand the Bible better than you ever have before ...

Find the answers you need!

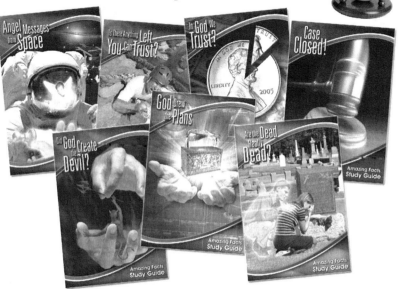

Send for the printed guides absolutely FREE!

✂ -

Bible Correspondence Course
P.O. Box 426
Coldwater, MI 49036

Name _____

Address _____

City _____

State _____ ZIP _____

Phone (____)_____ Email _____

Free offer available in North America and U.S. territories only.

GHL 08-13

The REMNANT STUDY BIBLE
WITH E.G. WHITE COMMENTS

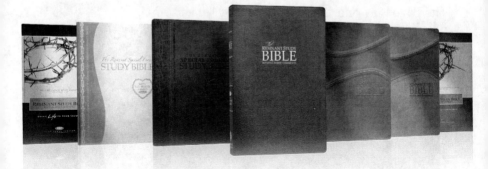

POWER-PACKED FEATURES

- Two-color Printing, Plus Words of Christ in Red Letter
- 20 Topical Studies Chained throughout the Bible with Index to Chains
- Thousands of Helpful End-of-verse Scripture Cross-References and Notes
- Full-Color Section Featuring Bible Timeline, Furniture and Cleansing of the Sanctuary, and Prophetic Symbols
- How to Use Section, Brief Biography of Ellen G. White, Bible Symbols and Their Meanings, Parables and Miracles of Jesus Christ, Read Your Bible through in a Year Guide, How Sin Began, and More
- Extensive Concordance, 8-page Section of Color Maps, 2 Ribbon Markers, Generous Margins, Plus Much More!

NEW KING JAMES VERSION

Genuine Cowhide
RP1059 **$99.95**

Leathersoft Brown and Black
RP1060 **$85.95**

Leathersoft Burgundy and Black
RP1061 **$85.95**

Leathersoft Special Forces Brown
RP1063 **$89.95**

Leathersoft Special Forces Lavender
RP1064 **$89.95**

Hardcover Edition
RP1085 **$49.95**

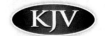

KING JAMES VERSION

Genuine Cowhide
RP1073 **$99.95**

Leathersoft Brown and Black
RP1074 **$85.95**

Leathersoft Burgundy and Black
RP1075 **$85.95**

Leathersoft Special Forces Brown
RP1076 **$89.95**

Leathersoft Special Forces Lavender
RP1077 **$89.95**

Hardcover Edition
RP1078 **$49.95**

CALL (800) 423-1319 OR VISIT: WWW.REMNANTPUBLICATIONS.COM

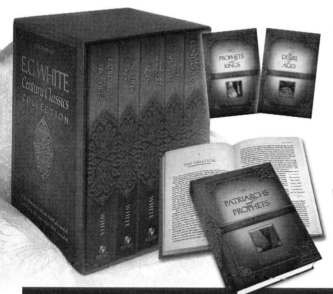
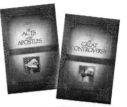

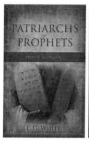 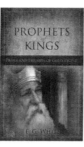 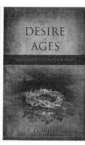 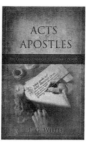 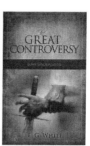